Pleasure from the Mister

Pleasure from the Mister

SEX SECRETS FOR UNBRIDLED PASSION INSPIRED BY THE BESTSELLING NOVEL

Marisa Bennett

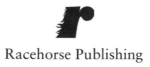

Racehorse Publishing

Copyright © 2019 by Hollan Publishing, Inc.

All Rights Reserved. No part of this book may be reproduced in any manner without the express written consent of the publisher, except in the case of brief excerpts in critical reviews or articles. All inquiries should be addressed to Skyhorse Publishing, 307 West 36th Street, 11th Floor, New York, NY 10018.

Racehorse Publishing books may be purchased in bulk at special discounts for sales promotion, corporate gifts, fund-raising, or educational purposes. Special editions can also be created to specifications. For details, contact the Special Sales Department, Skyhorse Publishing, 307 West 36th Street, 11th Floor, New York, NY 10018 or info@skyhorsepublishing.com.

Racehorse Publishing™ is a pending trademark of Skyhorse Publishing, Inc.®, a Delaware corporation.

Visit our website at www.skyhorsepublishing.com.

10 9 8 7 6 5 4 3 2 1

Library of Congress Cataloging-in-Publication Data is available on file.

Print ISBN: 978-1-63158-539-5
E-Book ISBN: 978-1-63158-540-1

Cover design by Brian Peterson

Printed in the United States of America

DEDICATION

To my very own Mister.

CONTENTS

INTRODUCTION

Take it from the Mister. What's found in fiery romance novels doesn't have to stay on the page. Let love or lust lead you down a pathway to passion, where your deepest fantasies become reality. You hold in your hands the secret window to brimming pleasure, where you can unlock your hidden desires or refresh the sexy sessions that need some attention. Whether your fancy is low-lit evenings with soft, sensual caresses; a good old-fashioned romp; or something a little naughtier; this bedside companion will give you options to pine for every day and night.

Unbutton a world of excitement as you explore all kinds of positions for your romantic, mouthy, and kinky play. Get swept off your feet or take the lead by sharing this book with your partner. As you pore over these pages and one another, you'll find heated opportunities to spice up your foreplay and your coreplay, to ask for what you want, and to bring each other to climactic heights.

Take a lesson in lust from the one who knows best, and get ready to reach peak passion in your own living romance.

"I want to do with you what spring does with the cherry trees."

—Pablo Neruda

Chapter One

Sweet Seductions

Romantic Play

While you and your partner may not recite Shakespearean sonnets as you gaze adoringly at one another (or do you?), there's something to be said for the kind of sex that gets you all tingly. After all, it's the reason why people fall in love and (purposely) procreate. These positions cater to the times when you want to show a little love and affection, lock eyes while you get intimate, or be touching as much of the person as you can possibly manage.

Hello, I Love You

Get snuggled up all close and personal for this sweet seductive position. It's a big crowd-pleaser, because the hot hip angle lets him go deep and sets her up for optimal clitoral stimulation. You both have control over the rhythm and depth of the thrusts, so you can take this position from a slow grind all the way up to a gallop, as your tryst takes off!

He sits in a chair. She sits in his lap, facing him, with her knees bent and placed on either side of his

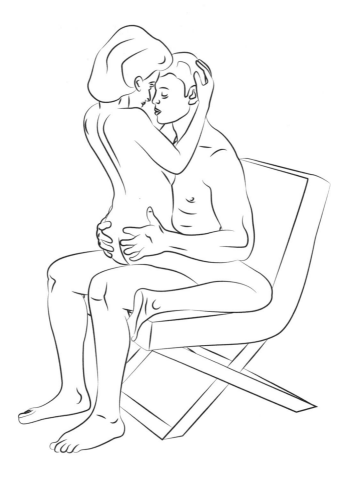

hips. Both partners have both hands free to roam around to show just how much they love what they do to each other.

When you're close enough to touch, take advantage of it: let your hands roam and explore your partner. Try touching your partner in new ways; let's be honest, we all tend to follow the same routines, and it's easy to hone into the same hot spots, but when you try this move, let your hands find some new ways to play.

IN THE HOT SEAT

No silly trivia questions for you in this hot seat, just some nice hot loving! Sitting interlocked with your partner, you're on equal footing. This position lets you each take charge controlling the rhythm and speed of your fun; you can even take turns!

He sits on the bed with his legs spread out in front of him. She sits between his legs, facing him, with her knees up and her feet outside of his hips. Both of them lean back on their hands as their eyes meet across the (un)crowded bedroom.

This position has you doing it face to face, but you're just out of reach for (comfortable) kissing. Instead, look your partner in the eye. Keeping eye contact during sex is incredibly intimate; so don't

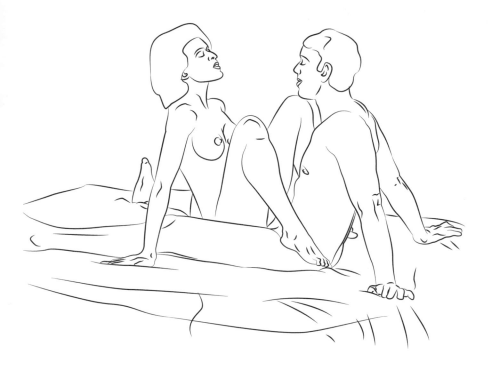

worry if it doesn't come naturally. Watching your partner can be enlightening as you watch their reactions to your movements and touches. We all like to playact a bit during sexy times, but you'll know your partner is enjoying herself when you can see it plainly on her face!

LOCK AND KEY

He's the key, and she's the lock—it's just one more phallic euphemism, or one more really bad pickup line. But believe me, this is one lock you'll both want to get open.

She lies on her side, top leg bent and rolled down to the mattress in front of her. He positions himself between her legs and enters her, his hands behind her back.

The key's got the easy job here: He has easy access and can slide right in. Spending too much time in this position is hard on the lock, and it could cause tension in her back or shoulders, so keep the massage oil handy! Still if you can stick it, this position is a big win. The unusual angle makes all the difference, since with her torso twisted, she's a snug fit! Sideways positions like this one are always good to mix into your repertoire, since they add one more

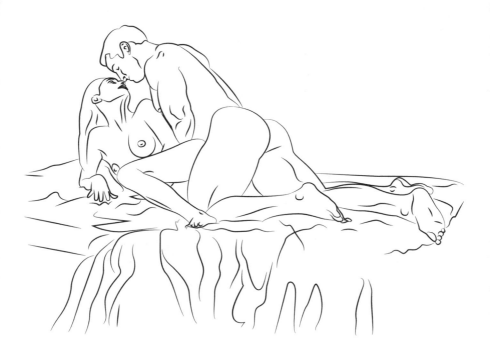

orientation to the "who's on top" question, and they typically give you a tight squeeze.

SWEET NOTHINGS

This position will have you doing it cheek-to-cheek, giving you a chance to whisper sweet words to one another (or naughty instructions!). The close contact and precipitous placement give this position a double dose of sexy, so you'll be dying to try this one again! Just be careful not to thrust your way off the bed and onto the floor—although I doubt the change in scenery will slow you down. . . .

She lies on the bed with her upper body off the bed supported by her arms (in a push-up stance). He positions himself between her legs, then stretches out on top of her, putting his hands on the floor next to hers. This position works because he supports most of his weight on his own arms, so her rib cage is not squashed beneath him.

For maximum thrusting power, and to keep her from freefalling forward, he may want to press her calves down with his ankles. That way he can brace himself against her for even deeper strokes. She can use her strong upper body to push back against him for double the friction if she wants to get into the fun!

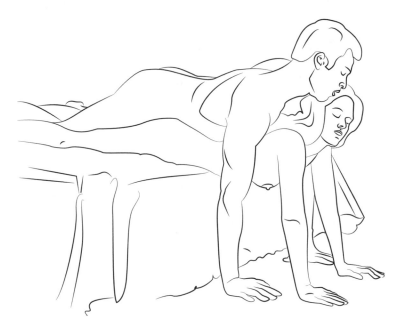

"No, the heart that has truly lov'd never forgets, But as truly loves on to the close; As the sunflower turns on her god when he sets The same look which she turn'd when he rose."

—Thomas Moore

Pillow Talk Dos and Don'ts

Bedroom dirty talk is one thing, but what do you say when you want to let your lover know you care? It's all "fuck me!" this and "oh don't stop!" that; what ever happened to a little romance? Here are some basic tips to help you say the right thing.

Do use the pet name you know your partner likes.

"Oh baby, you know I love what you do to me!"

Don't use pet names you just came up with. I know it seemed like a good idea at the time, but . . .

"Oh YES, you're so GOOD my Ass Queen!"

Do give instructions to help them hit the right spot.

"Yes! Touch me there, softer!"

Don't give critiques.

"You really need to tighten up your tongue technique down there, guy!"

Do check in.
"Do you like that, huh, baby?"

Don't zone out.

"Huh? What was that, hon? I was watching the weather."

Do try new things.

"Guess what new toy just came in the mail!?"

Don't try new things before talking it over!

"What, you didn't like my new strap-on?"

Do tell him or her what you're planning.

"I'm going to flip you over and ride you until you come!"

Don't talk about weekend plans.
"We need to get the car inspected this weekend, but we can do that on the way to my parents' house. . . . "

STAND AND DELIVER

This move helps you make the fantasy of wild sex standing up a bit more doable! With a little leg up from your furniture and a bit of upper-body strength, you'll be on your way to vertical nirvana. Since your hands will be busy keeping you up, use the rest of your body to control the action. Small movements or adjustments—maybe a tilt of your hips?—can make a big difference in this position.

He stands by the edge of the bed. She wraps her arms around him and lifts her legs onto the bed with one foot on either side of him. He uses one arm to hold her closer to him with the other hand under her thigh to give her a bit more support. She can brace her legs against the bed to raise and lower herself against him (while he tries to stay upright!).

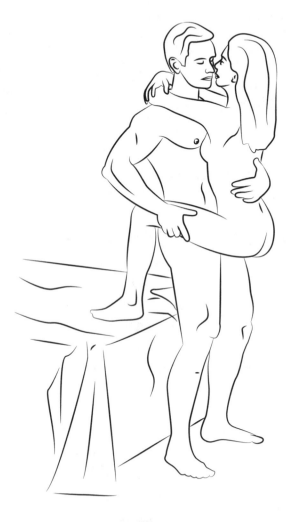

"Then fly betimes, for only they conquer love that run away."

—Thomas Carew

This position makes good use of normal bedroom scenery to get things done! Keep that in mind when you're trying this one out; if your bedroom has a more convenient arrangement, use that to your advantage. Walls can be very helpful here: if your bed is by the wall, you can try this position in the space between the bed and the wall. She still rests her feet on the bed, but he turns to lean her back against the wall. This way he has even more support to hold her up, so they can keep going for longer—and with the extra support, you'll both have better leverage for deeper thrusts that hit just the right spot!

Chapter Two

Twisted Trysts

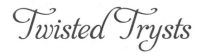

Stepping it Up

*I*f you put your leg on the blue dot, and I put mine on the yellow. . . . Trying to have sex like you're competing for a Twister championship can get a little tricky. Thankfully, it usually pays off, whether because you've managed to find the right combination of flailing legs and arms, or because screwing it up and falling off the bed is just as fun as being a sommelier of bendy sex. These moves are all twisty fun, so get in touch with your inner salted pretzel and try out these tantric tangles.

All Tangled Up

Like vines of ivy winding along a brick wall, this position makes it difficult to tell where one ends and the other begins.

This position is most easily begun in a spooning position, with her being the little spoon. She should turn to lie mostly flat on her back, while he brings his upper leg in between hers. Her upper leg should be lifted to give him enough space to insert himself from

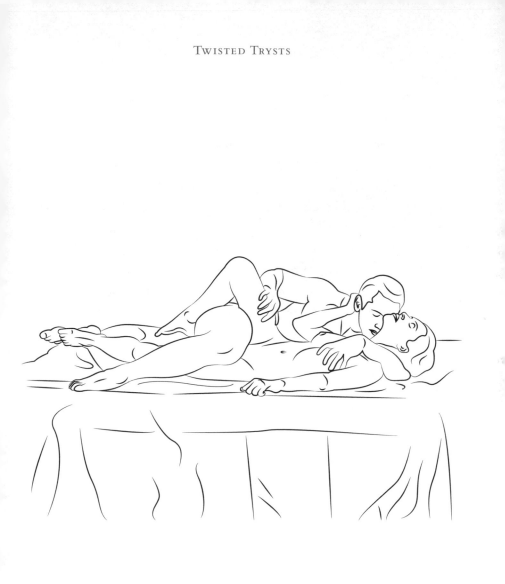

behind, and her knees should be bent over his leg so that she can use it to help her thrust. Their intertwining legs will make for a slower, more sensual pace where both partners can glide along each other. Since her upper body is still laying flat, he can still lean in and nibble at her ears, kiss her neck, or move in for a steamy make out. He can use his upper arm to linger a soft hand along her legs, tease her clitoris, or hold on to her hips. In the meantime, his lower arm can be under her to support her head, and the free hand is in perfect range to cup and massage her breast.

Get all tangled up with your partner, whether it's in the sheets or in a patch of ivy (just make sure it's not poisoned).

PIN-UP GIRL

Half the fun of sex is being able to watch how sexy your partner looks while you get down and dirty with each other. This position has her demurely poised for him for that classically sexy look of the pin-up generation.

No acrobatics required! This one has her lying down on the bed, floor, or basically any other surface you don't mind having sex on. He kneels in

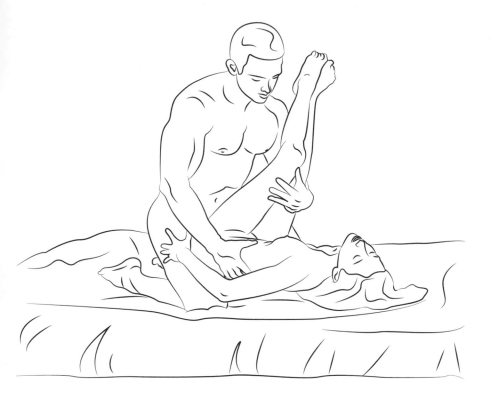

front of her, while she scoots her butt to meet him. Both of her legs should be raised, but this one isn't a flexibility contest. Her legs can be bent comfortably, and pivoted slightly to one side so they rest on his shoulder. He can support her legs with one hand, while he guides her hips with the other. This position has her lying comfortably out on the bed, which will give him access to her breasts, and the ability to gauge her facial expressions (otherwise known as her I'm-Almost-There!-O-Meter). Keeping her legs together will make it a nice, tight fit, and the angle of her raised hips will bring him deeper inside her.

This position is incredibly easy, but a classic for a reason!

SHIPS PASSING IN THE NIGHT

Not every position has to feel like only a contortionist could do it. For those of us who like to try out new angles—hold the torn ligament—this one is just right.

Both partners should lie down on the bed parallel to one another, facing the same side of the room. His head should be at her feet, and her feet should be at his head. He should enter her from behind, and if necessary, her body can be angled in a slight L in order

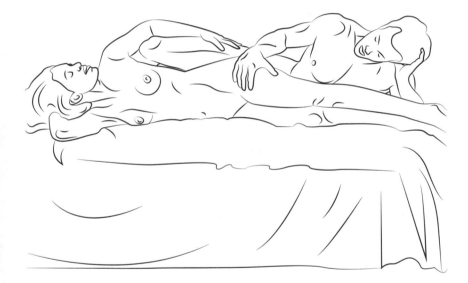

to let him in more easily. This position isn't the crazy-sex-hair-giving kind. It mostly stays at a slow, sensual pace, where both partners can caress and tease one another, working up to a slow, long climax. He can tease her clitoris, and she can reach a hand between his legs to massage his balls.

Be careful not to get too comfy, though—nobody likes it when a partner falls asleep on the job!

REVERSE COWBOY

Everyone knows how much fun reverse cowgirl can be, but what about a little reverse action for him? This position puts him in charge of the lasso, and it's her who gets taken for a ride.

This one requires some furniture that can handle a good romp. It works best with a comfortable chair and an ottoman, but a couch can be substituted. Since this position is a little nontraditional, he may not be used to putting his penis in from an upside down position. Giving her some warm-up cunnilingus or sensual foreplay will make it a lot easier for him to slip in when it's time to get rolling. She should sit back in her favorite chair, with her legs extended onto the ottoman in front of her. He should straddle her, facing

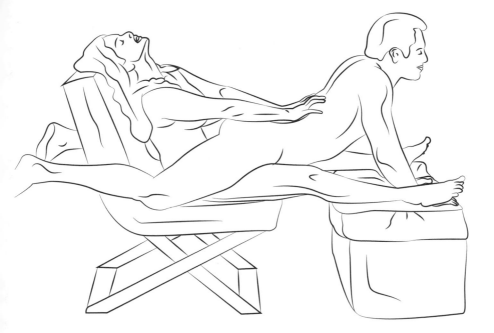

away, using the ottoman in front of him for support. The chair works best here because his legs can lie flat behind it, whereas with a couch he'll have to bend his legs up and have less space to move. The tricky part is making the entrance. She should keep her legs wide while he faces his pelvis down and forward while he goes in. Once this has happened, it's a lot easier to keep in sync. She gets a rarely seen view of his butt, and he gets to feel her from a whole new angle.

Jigsaw Puzzle

Putting together a puzzle on a rainy day is a great way to keep your mind sharp. But for sunny days, hazy days, or days that end in Y, putting together those penis and vagina puzzles keeps everything else sharp.

She lies down perpendicularly across a chair. She should bring her knees to her chest to make room for him to join the puzzle. From there, he should squat down, facing away, and angle his hips forward so that he can enter her from above. She can rest her legs on his back, which is a convenient lounging position for her, and will also keep things nice and tight for him. This position is particularly fun, because, hey!

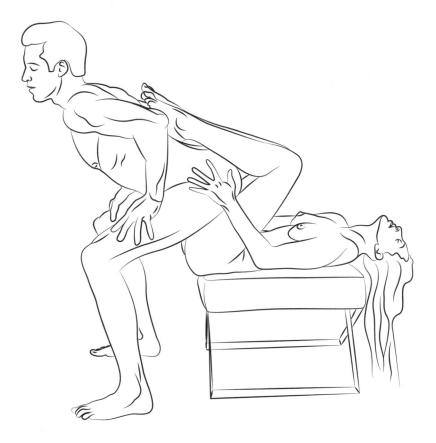

His penis is upside down! The flip-flopping of sexy parts will give attention to all sorts of sensitive zones that traditional sex doesn't usually hit. Because of the angle, he'll also surprise her with a steady rhythm of pressure from his balls on her clitoris as he pumps away.

Adding a little human Tetris to your repertoire is the best way to figure out how you fit together!

MODERN DANCE

You don't need a background in ballet to make your sexy sessions look like *Swan Lake*. With a little upper body strength from him, and some leg extensions from her, your next rendezvous will be the best choreography yet!

She should lie on her side on the edge of the bed, so that her hips come to the edge. He stands at the edge of the bed, facing forward. After she straightens her leg so that her toes point to the ceiling, he should take hold of her thigh, and bring it close to his chest so that her leg extends beyond his shoulders. With his other hand, he can support her bum or hips. She should use her elbow to keep her torso lifted off the bed. Her other leg should be comfortably folded in

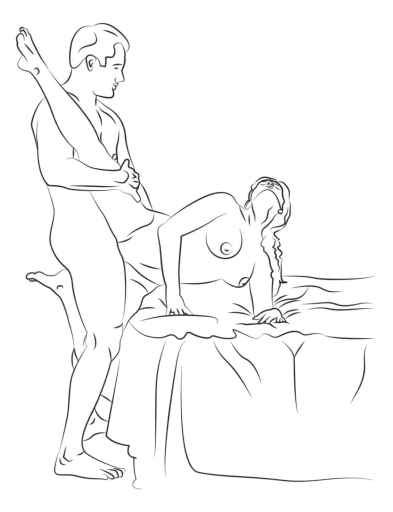

between his legs. She should use her arms to push up from the bed every time he pulls her up in a lusty thrust.

This position requires a lot of upper body strength from both partners, but is worth it because of how deeply he can penetrate her, and because it explores the highly underrated sideways entrance.

THE TURNTABLE

There's a little bit of a DJ in all of us. Whether you want to do the spinning, or you want your record spun, this hot take on sideways loving will give your trysts a new remix.

She lies down on the bed, bringing her knees to her chest. Her feet should be up in the air, but they don't need to be spread far apart. Instead of lying directly on top of her, he should angle himself perpendicularly over her. Entering her sideways gives both of them a tight squeeze and she can make him even more snug inside by tightening her thighs together. She can continue to alter the sensations by leaning her closed legs to one side or another.

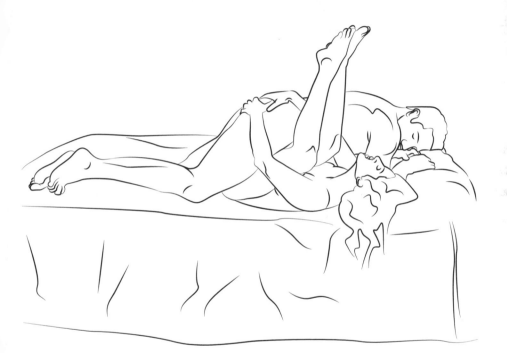

This position gives him creative control over the pace and rhythm of the encounter, while she gets to lie back and feel him work.

PRIM AND PROPER

A good girl should always keep her legs crossed. This position lets her be a good girl while she does bad girl things!

She lies down on the bed, with him on his knees directly in front of her. She should cross her legs so that her right foot rests on his right shoulder, and her left foot rests on his left shoulder. He can hold on to either her ankles or knees to keep her in place. She can cross her legs by her shins, or for a tighter fit, cross above the knee. Changing where her legs are crossed throughout this lusty session will keep things interesting. This is a great angle for both partners to watch each other work as things get steamy.

Though he is in the most control in this position, she doesn't have to just lay back and hang out. She can squeeze her PC muscles to help make a pulsing, tighter sensation around his shaft, or if she wants to give him a good show, tease her own nipples and squeeze her breasts every time his motions have made an especially good impact!

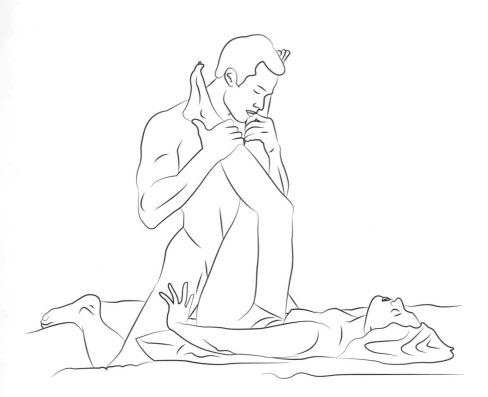

"Thus if men and women act according to each other's liking, their love for each other will not be lessened even in one hundred years."

—*The Kama Sutra*

"Ye Gods! annihilate
but space and time,
And make two lovers
happy."

—Alexander Pope

⌇

IS THAT YOUR LEG OR MINE?

There are some positions that you try because you're feeling acrobatic, some because of yoga, and others that happen because in all that rolling around, you've managed to get tangled into one big, sensational feeling jumble. This is one of those!

He lies down on the bed with his knees up and feet raised slightly in the air. She faces away, crouching down over his pelvis with her feet flat on the bed and her knees up. Instead of keeping both of her feet in between his legs, she should have one leg between his legs, and the other straddled over his right leg (or left, if she's a lefty). Her hips should face the thigh she is straddling. Because his legs are perched a little bit off the bed, his upper thigh will graze her clitoris as she takes the reins of this twisty dynamic. He has free hands to fondle as he pleases, while she can use her hands to either guide herself up and down, or cup and massage his balls as she goes.

In this leggy tryst, she's in the captain's chair. The angles of both partners' hips are perfect for extra-deep penetration, and his tangled legs against her sensitive spots will keep her dedicated to getting him there.

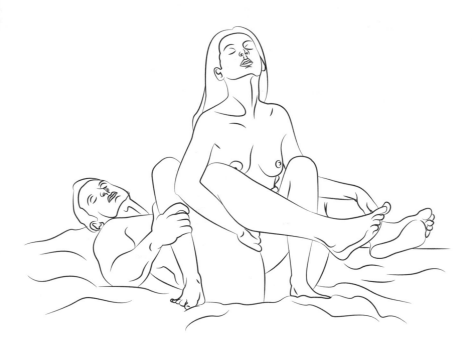

NAUGHTY ROLL-UP

If regular 69ing has got you down (since, you know, being upside down on someone while you simultaneously perform and receive mind-blowing head is so boring), try out the naughty version!

This one requires a little bit of flexibility from her, so make sure she stretches first! She lies down on the bed, and raises her legs in the air, as parallel to her own head as possible. If she can clasp on to her ankles with straightened legs, woohoo! If not, she's like the other 90 percent of the population without a PhD in Being Bendy, and that's totally fine. Holding on to the backs of her knees works too. He should kneel over her, so that his penis is accessible to her mouth without her having to do much of anything. With his arms on either side of her hips, or grasping her bum, he should be face to face with her sweet spot.

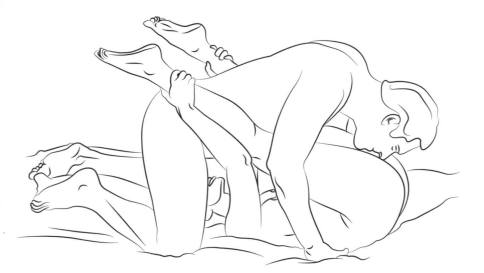

This is where roads diverge. This position is spectacular for giving and receiving some good old-fashioned fellatio, but it also gives the opportunity for some backdoor attention. If you and your partner are comfortable, try letting your tongue explore some new places. Your front end isn't the only place packed with nerves ready to be teased! If not, being curled up in a ball while you 69 is still pretty effing sexy. Everyone wins!

Be forward thinking and try out this role-reversal!

Chapter Three

Pleasuring Her Orally

DOWN TO GO DOWN

c2~

P enetrative sex is a crapshoot for women. Studies show that only 25 percent of women regularly orgasm from penetration, which means that a majority of ladies are putting out and not getting much in return. At least, not from p-in-the-v sex. But with oral, it's different: the focus is on her, and she's much more likely to get off. Women's orgasms are amazing: where male orgasms tend to last 6 seconds, an average female orgasm lasts 20 seconds, and most women can have multiple orgasms in a single romp! Going down, eating out, cunnilingus, whatever you call it, oral sex is an intimate experience: you're face to face with a part of her very few people get to be intimately acquainted with.

WHAT'S UP DOWN THERE: A GUIDE TO LADYBITS ANATOMY

c2~

Before you get down, you should take a look at where you're going. Whether you're a native of vagina-land or a backpacking visitor (or even a new tourist! Welcome!), it's worth it to take a look at the map. While we normally use the word "vagina" to talk about the whole ladybits ecosystem, technically "vagina" only refers to the vaginal opening. That's a serious misnomer, since the vagina is such a small part of a woman's whole sexual experience; while it may be the star of the show in penetrative sex, if you want to really please a woman, you don't need to go deeper, you want to spread out! The word "vagina" comes from the Latin word for sheath—you know, the place where you put your sword. But anyone with a good sword-holder between her legs can tell you there's more to going down there than just the female end of an electrical socket.

The right term for the kit and caboodle is "vulva," a vaguely foreign word (try it with a Russian accent) that has potential for sexiness, although since it's not often used colloquially it still has the ring of a medical term. Women's vulvas are very different, which can create plenty of insecurity for anyone who doesn't look quite like the diagram in her health class text-book. Like snowflakes, no two pussies are exactly the same, but they all share the same basic parts that you should get to know.

LABIA MAJORA
(THE OUTER PUSSY LIPS)

I love the neat organization of the vulva, almost like someone has sorted the ladybits into charming little pink folders for easy access. The outermost "folder" is called the *labia majora*, literally the "big lips." The outer skin varies in sensitivity, but it can often be more receptive than you would think, when you consider how many women have their outer labia doused in wax and the hair ripped out!

The outer labia are physiologically similar to the scrotum, but don't expect it to be as delicate as a set of balls: your mileage may vary, but many women enjoy having their lips stroked, massaged, kissed, rubbed and otherwise played with during pussy play. As always be gentle and follow her lead!

LABIA MINORA
(THE INNER PUSSY LIPS)

The inner folder, tucked neatly inside the outer lips, is called the *labia minora*. These folds are softer and more sensitive than her outer lips: they are some-times called "nymphae," which I think is just lovely. The labia minora can look quite different from one woman to another, with some bigger or smaller, and varying in coloring. The inner lips also change in appearance when the woman is aroused, usually becoming larger and either darker or brighter (think "rosier") in color as blood rushes to the area. Because these inner lips are more sensitive than the outer lips, your attentions will likely be rewarded if you gently

lick, suck, and kiss all around here, paying attention to her responses. One good move is to slowly
trace a line from her vagina up to the spot just below
her clit, moving your tongue (or your wet or lubed
finger) between her pussy lips, parting them as you
go. This is a nice teasing move that helps you gauge
her response. Does she try to move you faster? Push
you up toward her clit? Sigh and lie back to enjoy
what you're doing? Pay attention and follow her lead
to give her the most pleasure!

CLITORIS

The love button. The little man in the boat. The
mysterious clit, only revealed to the most astute
and attentive lover—well, let's hope not, because if
she wants to come, then you should be intimately
acquainted with her clitoris.

First, an introduction: The clitoris is a mass of
nerve endings set right above the vagina, neatly tucked
beneath where the left and right lips of the labia minora
meet up, under a fold of skin called the clitoral hood.

The clitoris has eight thousand nerve endings, twice as many as are in the penis, all bundled
up together. But the clit you see is just the tip of
the iceberg. The visible clitoris is called the *glans
clitoris* (like the glans or head of a penis), and it is
the head of a larger system that branches out and

down toward the vagina. This theory accounts for the sometimes elusive g-spot, thought to be part of this network of nerves.

So the little clit is not to be ignored. But as Monty Python opined, "Why not start her off with a nice kiss? You don't have to go leaping straight for the clitoris like a bull at a gate." Aside from the fact that no one should be approaching the clitoris in any way that is bull-like, the point is that her clitoris is not an "on switch," and if you keep flicking it like that you're going to get punched in the face.

Even if a woman loves it when you rub her clit, your best bet is to start out with indirect stimulation and save rougher, more direct stimulation for when she's close to climax. There are plenty of ways for you to do this: licking and fondling her inner lips, working your way toward her clit. You can gently pull and tug on her pussy to make her clit rub up against the hood. You can even lick and fondle the hood itself for a closer indirect hit.

Once all systems are go and she's deep in a groove, you should switch it up a lot to see what seems to turn her on the most. But once she's indicated (through moans, screams, or by direct physical signs like pulling your hair or pushing you into her crotch) that you've gotten it *just right, that's it, right there*, then do a girl a favor and keep doing exactly what you're doing until she comes!

VAGINA

Vaginas are amazing, flexible, versatile things. They can stretch and squeeze to accommodate anything from a baby to a penis to a dildo—even an entire fist, if you're into that. And only with lube. Since there are fewer supersensitive nerve endings in and around the vagina than there are up by the clitoris, you don't want to focus all of your attentions there. Approach with caution the idea of "tongue-fucking" her: that move may be sexier in theory than actual practice, although your mileage may vary. Still, try adding a few fingers while you're focusing on her more sensitive spots, and she's in for a ride!

G-SPOT

When you're adding a few fingers, you should aim them in the direction of the g-spot, on the front wall of the vagina. This spot was named for Ernst Gräfenberg, and researchers have been studying and arguing about it since the 1600s. They're still arguing about it today: in 2009, British researchers conducting a questionnaire survey concluded that the g-spot did not exist, but more recent French experiments taking ultrasounds of women having sex have shown good evidence that the sensitive area exists, and changes while she's having sex. If you can't find it, don't be too concerned; just like any other move, this one works for some and not for others. But if you're exploring, try stroking the inside of her vagina, on the front wall about two inches in. Feel for an area with a rougher texture, and when you find it apply gentle pressure as you stroke. You can do this with the patented "come hither" wiggle, or make up your own technique!

OUT-OF-THIS-WORLD CUNNILINGUS POSITIONS

THE ROYAL DINNER

This position is fit for a queen, all she has to do is lie back and let you do the work. Think of it as the missionary position of cunnilingus, the go-to starter move, and for good reason! At this angle as your mouth is focused on her clitoris, you have very easy access to her vagina, and she's in the perfect position for you to stroke her g-spot.

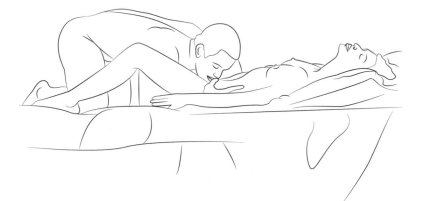

SHE'S ON TOP

Propped up on top, straddling your face, she has lots of control over the action. Lie on the bed and have her climb on top of you. Have her straddle your face, spreading her legs until she's lowered into place. She can stay on all fours or lean down on your torso, however is most comfortable. You get a new perspective, and a great view of her ass as you practice all your tricks. Follow her rhythm as she grinds against your mouth.

From this position your hands are free to roam. Use them to grip her hips and pull her closer, or squeeze her ass. She can also move freely: she can move closer to or farther from your mouth, or pull away if it gets too intense, coming back when she's ready.

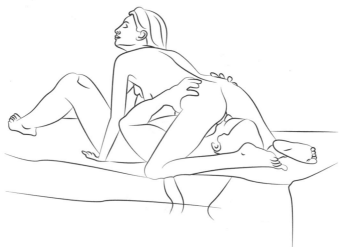

THREE-RING CUNNILINGUS

An exercise ball can add a fun balancing element to
your oral play: if you have one handy, try this move.
Or maybe it will inspire you to take up whatever
exercises you're *supposed* to do on an exercise ball.
Have her sit on the ball as you kneel in front of her.
Rest her legs on your shoulders as you bring your
face closer to her pussy. She can lean back and place
her hands on the ball to brace herself, while you hold
her hips to steady her and hold her close. She can
bounce, thrust, and sway, using the gentle motion of
the ball to give her another layer of sensation as you
work your own magic.

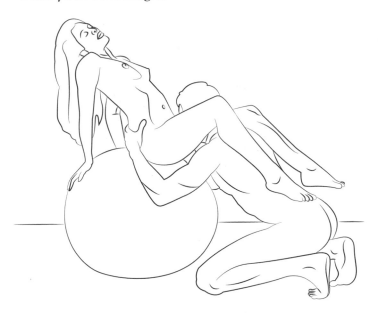

If you don't have an exercise ball, try cunnilingus with her seated on a chair or on the edge of the bed, with you kneeling between her legs. The angle of this position puts more focus on the clitoris, and gives your partner plenty of opportunity to participate: she can move her hips to redirect your tongue, shift herself to set the rhythm, and if the spirit moves her, she can grab your head to directly increase the pressure! She's also got a great view of the show!

STANDING OVATION

Good oral sex doesn't have to be horizontal: try this hot wall position when she wants to stretch her legs! Have her stand against a wall with her legs spread as wide as is comfortable. Arrange yourself between her legs: depending on your height, sit or kneel so your face is directly at pussy level. Move in close and wrap your hands around her hips and thighs to help steady her. Stroke, squeeze, and fondle her ass and legs as you go down on her. She can play with her tits, grip your head, or stand back and enjoy. This position is perfect for shower sex, as long as she can stay steady on her feet!

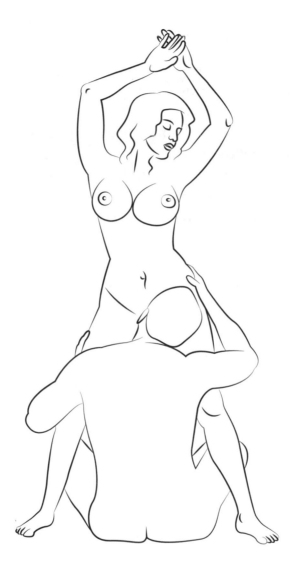

HULA GIRL

Can your girl spin a hula hoop? This position will have her moving her hips in no time! Recline on the edge of the bed, with your head hanging off. Have her stand at the foot of the bed, facing toward you, straddling your face. Have her move until she's in position while you help steady her with your hands. With her spread out above you, you have perfect access. She can shift her body to help you hit the right spot, and she has a great view of your work. Standing above you can help her feel in control: add some bondage, and you have a great scene for a starter dominatrix. Or maybe she just likes to hula!

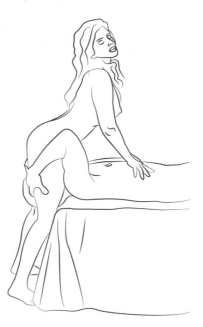

NO-HAND HANDSTAND

If you want a challenge with an explosive reward, try this acrobatic position. Pick her up and hold her against you, facing away. She can wrap her arms back and around you for extra stability, but you really shouldn't be trying this if you think you'll drop her on her head! If you can manage it, the flipped orientation makes this position super stimulating.

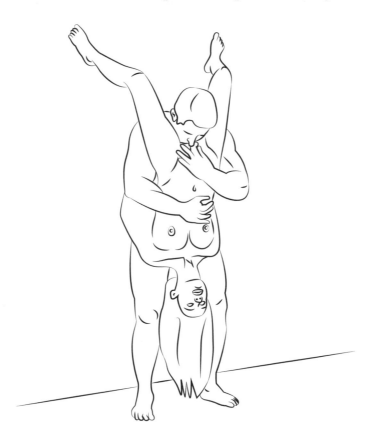

If you're not quite ready to join Cirque du Sex, don't despair: this position can be easily modified into a kind of intermediate free-weights move. Have her lie back across an ottoman or a big pillow—anything big enough to prop under her and make her arch her back. Have her hang her ass off the edge of it. Set yourself up between her legs, then slide your arms under her thighs and grab her ass. Lift her up to meet your mouth and give her your best moves, then lower her down, squeezing and massaging her ass. Then do as many reps as you can!

Chapter Four

Pleasuring Him Orally

As the apple tree among the trees of the forest, so is my beloved among the men. With great delight I sat in his shadow, and his fruit was sweet to my taste.

—Song of Solomon 2:3

Head of the Pack

ℭ

*A*ll men love head, therefore all men love
all head. False! Wrong! For the love of
God, just stop. It is a rare man who will
turn down fellatio, but there is more to giving
great head than just gracing his penis with your
presence. Whether going down is foreplay, coreplay,
or both for you and your partner, it's important to
know where you're going, where you want to take
him, and how you plan to get there. With a quick
brush-up on his anatomy, an ode to grooming, some
kink, and of course the how-to, this section will go
well beyond the need-to-knows of oral sex for him.
Your downtown dexterity (and enthusiasm!) will be
the difference between your guy just loving head—
and your guy loving *your* head.

What's Up Down There:
A Guide to Man Parts Anatomy

ℭ

All too often, the penis is given all of the attention,
while other zones that are just yearning to be touched,
licked, teased, and sucked are neglected. Here is a list

of some of the obvious and not-so-obvious zones of his manhood so that you can touch him in ways he'll fantasize about well after you've finished.

THE PENIS

This is your first problem: focussing on "the penis." His shaft is by no means one-dimensional (that would be a shame), both in terms of what he feels and how he feels it. So why do we talk about it as if it's a singular entity? All parts of the penis are not created equal, and as such, each part should be treated with special attention!

GLANS

The *glans*, coming from the Latin word for "acorn," is the rounded tip of the penis through which men both urinate and ejaculate. In uncircumcised men, the glans is covered by the foreskin unless he is aroused. Whether your guy is circumcised or not, this is the most sensitive area of the penis, and therefore a part you should learn to know and love. Referring to it as the "glans" may sound a tad medical while you're talking about getting someone off, so society has presented us with all sorts of nicknames throughout the years: "mushroom tip," "head," "helmet," and "dome," just to name a few.

Like the beacon of a lighthouse signaling sailors in the night, the tip of his penis is a beacon for bliss that you're meant to pay attention to. Use your tongue to flick rhythmically against the head or massage sensuously. Vary your pace, and while you work your magic elsewhere, feel free to massage it with your lubricated hand to keep his tantric tempo way up. While this hot spot is the equivalent of the clitoris in its sensitivity to all that attention you're giving it, keep in mind that giving it *too* much attention can occasionally go awry. Just like any sensitive zone, unpleasant textures, dryness, and too much friction can be painful. While some people joke that "just the tip" doesn't qualify for having had sex, the same can be said for giving phenomenal head. Be good to the tip, but don't forget that this is just one of the stops (and not necessarily the first) on the road to oral ecstasy.

CORONA

Aptly named after the Spanish word for "crown," the *corona* is the rounded ridge where the head of his penis meets the shaft. As the circumference of the *glans*, the corona is packed with sensitive nerves that are ready to be teased and tempted by your tongue.

Use the tip of your tongue to run along this sensitive ring or flick rapidly to keep him on high alert.

This is a good area to tease lightly before you take him in your mouth, as well as an excellent go-to if you've been concentrating on one area for too long. While it's important to have a steady rhythm as you go down on him, switching things up will keep things from getting monotonous.

MEATUS

The *meatus* is the hole in the center of the tip of his penis. It's a little-known pleasure zone, that with some added pressure with your tongue, will add a little something extra to your repertoire. Keep in mind, though, that while it's a uniquely good feeling, it's no El Dorado of hot spots—spending lengths of time here poking your tongue at it will just be confusing for everyone.

FRENULUM

The *frenulum* is the small bulb of flesh right below his corona, connecting to the shaft of the penis. This tiny cluster of nerves is so rich with pleasure potential that it's a shame it's often overlooked. When you're tonguing down his shaft and head, take a moment to run your tongue along the circumference of his tip, and then flick rapidly on the frenulum. If you think you've done too much "flicking" as it is, put your lips at the bottom of his shaft, lightly gather the soft layer of skin with your lips and teeth (no biting!) using a little bit of suction, and glide your way up to his frenulum, continuing to suck lightly as you go. End this with a sensual kiss to the head of his penis before you make your next move.

FORESKIN

If the man in your life is uncircumcised, then you are familiar with his *foreskin*. This is the soft sheath of skin that covers and protects the *glans* when the penis is not erect. It is also a mucous membrane, much like the inside of an eyelid. When the penis is erect, the foreskin glides back over the penis to reveal the head.

Circumcision is popular in western culture, both for religious and health reasons. In the Book of Genesis (17: 10-14), Abraham instructs men to be circumcised and to have their newborn boys circumcised. As a result, circumcision has become one of the first celebrations for a newborn in Jewish families. On the eighth day after a baby boy is born, families celebrate the *brit milah* (pronounced "bris milôh" or just "bris"). The newborn is circumcised by a medically trained *mohel* (male) or a *mohelet* (female). While circumcision is not synonymous with Christian practices, New Year's Day is the holy day *Feast of the Circumcision of Christ* (according to the

Semitic calculation of days). In the Christian faith, this day accounts for the first drop of blood that Jesus shed for humanity.

In secular western culture, circumcision is generally performed to deter some of the health risks that can (but not always) come along with foreskin. The moist ecosystem under the foreskin can facilitate the spread of sexually transmitted diseases. However, and this is a big *however*, using protection and being a generally sanitary person about man care substantially decreases any of these risks, just as it would for a circumcised man.

While some talking (helmeted) heads like to argue that circumcision *is just so terrible! How dare you suggest I remove things from my amazing penis and subject me to a world devoid of pleasure!!!*, this is mostly just hubbub. There is no medical evidence to suggest that circumcision, when done properly, is harmful or negatively affects the penis's sensitivity. While much of this information seems like a cheerleading session for circumcision, many lovers of the uncircumcised man prefer the foreskin for its texture—the ribbed sensation along his penis can make it feel like he's doing two things at once while you're getting down and dirty.

Whether your partner is circumcised or un-, performing fellatio is generally the same in terms of your tantalizing technique. As long as you are paying attention to your partner's *oohs* and *ahhs*, the sheath doesn't affect his sword. Either way, there should be no stigma regarding the haves and have-nots, because penises are wonderful.

SCROTUM

Ohhhh, the *scrotum*! This should be one of your very favorite parts of the entire head-giving process, especially because it's one of his. The scrotum is the soft sack of skin that is the mahogany treasure chest to his family jewels. This area is extremely sensitive, both on the surface of his skin and on the sperm-producing testes themselves.

Get ready to lick, suck, massage and tease this area. If taking his balls into your mouth isn't your thing, you should really reconsider. If you've reconsidered, asked the heavens, spoken with oracles, and summoned an old shaman to find peace with the term "teabagging," and it's *still* not your thing, then just make sure to substitute the pleasure he would feel from your warm and wet mouth over him with your lubricated warm hands instead. The slippery sensation over his balls and sack while you give him head will have him writhing in ecstasy.

SCROTAL RAPHE

The *scrotal raphe* is the formation in the center of the skin of his balls that looks like a seam. The "raphe" is a term used for several different parts of the body, like the *lingual raphe*, which is the seam of skin on the underside of the tongue.

His nether raphe—not unlike the rest of his balls—is supersensitive and craves its own oral attention. While you're down there, think of the raphe as a line from point A to point Bliss: using the raphe as a guide, run your moistened tongue from the very bottom of his balls along this pleasure line, all the way up to the bottom of his penis. The sensation of your tongue running along this line will have him trembling as he gets ready for more attention from you and your mouth.

PERINEUM

Just behind the scrotum and right before you get to his back end, the *perineum* is the soft space in between. Sometimes referred to as the "gooch" or the "taint" (because t'aint your ass and t'aint your genitalia), the perineum's hypersensitivity is unsurprising, as it connects two major erogenous zones: his package and his back door. This spot is often neglected, but it is brimming with euphoric potential.

One mistake oral novices make is not getting handsy or exploratory enough. Yes, you are performing a blow job, which inherently implies mouth-to-penis action. But skipping over the less conspicuous bliss spots would be a mistake—like only hitting the major tourist hubs while you're on vacation and missing the hidden local gems. Gently massage his perineum while performing oral, or get even saucier and use your mouth. Take his penis in your mouth to lubricate his shaft, and then continue to massage it with your hand or massage his balls while you tongue his perineum. This technique borders on the seriously naughty because it's just shy of his back end, which is suggestive of a whole other world of deep desires.

ANUS

Yup, the butthole; how sexy for you! While many are adverse to the idea, incorporating his back door is one of those earth-shattering things that will change his perspective on head forever. With regards to female anatomy, there is no secret g-spot back there that is guaranteed to make a woman come, other than indirect clitoral stimulation. Luckily for men, such a pleasure hub exists! The prostate glands are located on the opposite side of the anal wall. Because of this, men can achieve orgasm from anal stimulation without even a stroke or a lick to the penis.

While you're performing fellatio, consider using your hands to sensually massage his balls, slowly move to his perineum, and then gently insert a lubricated finger into his anus. Multitasking is important, because for the man who wants his partner to explore anal play but may not want to address it, having your mouth on his cock at the same time is a good enough excuse for why he's moaning, *Holy shit, [your name here], that's so fucking good!* This form of anal playtime is generally a last-stop-on-the-road technique before you expect him to come (which he'll do, explosively), and one that should be performed by your non-dominant hand to avoid any cross-contamination.

OUT-OF-THIS-WORLD BLOW-JOB POSITIONS

cᒄ

THE HANDSTAND

You sexy acrobats, you! This position requires extensive balance and upper body strength by him, and the ability to stand by you. While he may be exerting exorbitant amounts of energy while you casually stand in front, the payoff for him is that—*oh right!*— he is getting his dick sucked. He should perform a steady handstand against a trusted wall (partitions made of rice paper with paintings of calming bonsai trees are not recommended), perhaps putting a soft mat on the floor to lessen the tension on his hands. Keep in mind that as you perform fellatio, his penis will be at the opposite angle to that of a traditional blow job. As you stand, lower your back and bring his penis upwards or kneel down to take his penis in your mouth from below. With such an open stance, he is presenting himself as a smooth canvas for you to kiss, lick, and massage without instruction or interference. By exerting so much energy and letting the blood rush to his head during this erotic blow job, he will let all-consuming sensations heighten the intensity he feels on his dick. Be wary of reaching a climax in this position, though, as it may weaken his arms and send him headfirst to the floor.

THE HOLY GRAIL

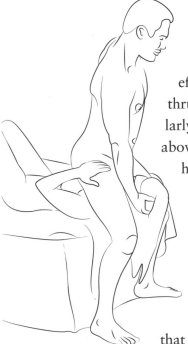

This position is a fellatio switch-eroo, which requires very little effort from you, and slow, erotic thrusting from him. Lie perpendicularly on the bed, while he straddles above you. Gently cupping your head and the back of your neck to prevent tension or strain, he performs *irrumatio*, which is essentially reverse fellatio. The term "fellatio" refers to you performing oral pleasure on a man, who remains passive, whereas "irrumatio" means that you are passive and the man performs the motions of oral sex. He should be sure to keep a slow, sensual pace, so as not to hurt or gag you. You can use your tongue and mouth to sensually lick and suck his penis as he glides in and out. At the same time, you can run your fingertips up and down his thighs, balls, backside, arms and chest to heighten his excitement. This position transforms a run-of-the-mill blow job into a sexy interactive event.

THE CROSSROADS

Meeting a crossroads doesn't have to be a life-changing event, but it can definitely change the way you think of giving phenomenal head. He lies down on the bed with his feet resting on the floor. You

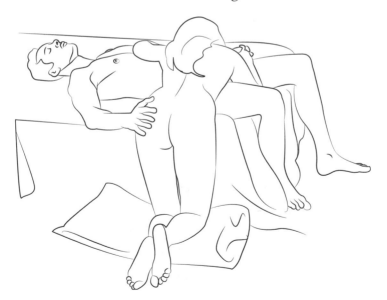

kneel on the floor perpendicularly to him (i.e., you should be facing the horizontal view of his abdomen). This angle allows your mouth to glide down his penis at a different angle from traditional fellatio, which will let your tongue explore those surfaces of his shaft that are needy for attention. This angle also gives you free rein to caress his legs and massage his balls, while presenting the opportunity for him to clutch your ass to ride along his pleasure trajectory.

TWO FOR ONE

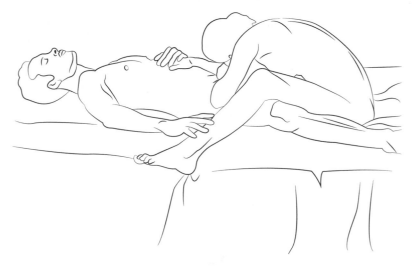

Oral sex doesn't have to be the main event; it should also be used as foreplay to make your lusty session all the more mind-blowing. In this position, he lies down on the bed as if you were performing traditional fellatio at his waist below. The difference here is that your legs straddle his hips so that you are at the ready to pounce on his dick when you so desire. This does require a little flexibility on your part, as you'll be slouched over his package as if you were trying to touch your nose to the floor at yoga. The great thing about this sexy straddle is that you get to take control and be a little selfish with your own pleasure needs. As you give him head and get him riled up, visualize what it'll feel like to be riding on top of him to get yourself hot and bothered. When you feel like joining the fun, spring up and slide yourself onto his shaft to ride each other into ecstasy. To add a kinky twist, switch back and forth between giving him head and fucking him; he'll think it's super hot that you're tasting your own flavor while you tongue him down.

BALL BLISS

Count giving your guy oral bliss as your exercise for the day! Using an exercise ball, have him sit centered on the ball as he awaits your oral gift. Kneel down between his legs, teasing him by running your fingers from the insides of his feet, around his ankles, and up the insides of his thighs. Follow this soft touch with your pouted lips and light, tonguey kisses. You'll be able to tell how well you're teasing him by how bouncy that ball starts to get. As you make your way to his package, lightly kiss the insides of his pelvis, bringing your tongue to his balls. While he controls the exercise ball, you'll control his: Lightly cradle his testicles with soft hands and take them into your mouth, being sure to move your tongue around them in a sensual massage. Quickly move from doing this to moistening his shaft with your mouth, and as you return to sucking his balls, massage his now-wet penis with your free hand. The two sensations at once will feel incredible for him and exciting for you as you watch his reaction. Just be careful—the more he likes it, the more the ball will bounce and potentially gag you (and you can save ballgags for another time!).

SOIXANTE-NEUF!

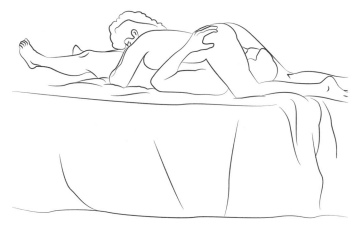

This is the most basic form of the 69 position, or soixante-neuf if you want to be all French about it. From this position both partners can rock their newly honed skills (you did just read the rest of this book, right?) at the same time! Position yourselves comfortably, so you can reach your partner easily and touch where you'll want to. If you're the lady on top, try to resist the urge to be up on your knees: you may need to lift up a little to accommodate different-sized partners, but try to keep your body close to his. This lets him apply a bit more pressure, and makes it a bit of a different up close encounter. While he's at work, she can go down on him from above. This angle makes it easier for her to deep-throat, but she can also use her mouth on the head of his cock while her fingers slide over the shaft.

Chapter Five
Old Dog, New Tricks

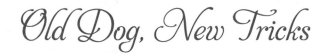

FROM–BEHIND FRONTRUNNING

R ear-entry sex has quite a reputation: like the guy in a leather jacket smoking a butt behind the school, positions like Doggie Style are hot because they feel so *bad*! There's nothing sweet or sensual about it—it's just unadulterated, animalistic sex. There's certainly something to be said for being bad, so why not give it a try? Whether you do it from behind standing up, laying down, or on all fours like Molly the golden retriever, this chapter has plenty of hot rear-entry positions to get your drag-racing motor running.

THE CHARIOT

Brush up on your Greek mythology and make your own Chariot of the Sun. Just don't lose control of it and incur the wrath of thunderbolt-hurling Zeus, because that would suck. This requires quite a bit of upper body strength from both partners, so doing fifty push-ups immediately before starting this position may not be the wisest choice if you want to make it last.

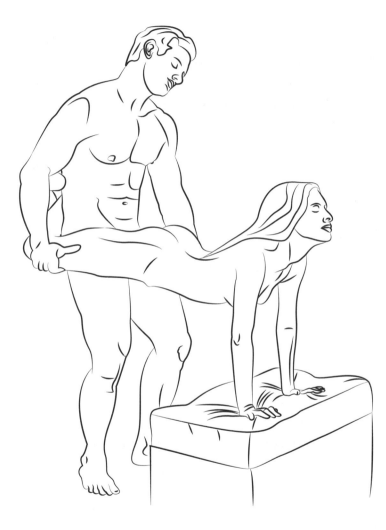

She places her hands flat on a chair or on the edge of the bed. Whatever piece of furniture is put in front of her, it needs to be sturdy (i.e., make sure it doesn't have wheels, lest she go flying). He stands behind her and slowly lifts her legs to his hips while she supports her upper body in a push-up move. As he enters her, she wraps her legs around his torso for extra stability.

This gravity-defying stunt is hard to pull off, but a thrill if you can get it right! If you have trouble lining everything up, try using different props of varying heights, like a tall chair or a lower bench. Once you've put everything together, you're ready to ride off to the Colosseum together!

CLOSING THE SUITCASE

Take the doggie-style position. Now rotate it about 90 degrees counterclockwise, and you get this hot girl-on-top rear-entry position that looks a bit odd, but feels AMAZING! So grab your passport, you've got a first-class ticket on the Orgasm Express!

This spin on the traditional doggie style lets her control the speed and depth of their thrusts while she uses his legs for support. He lies back on a bench or on the edge of the bed and draws his knees up to his

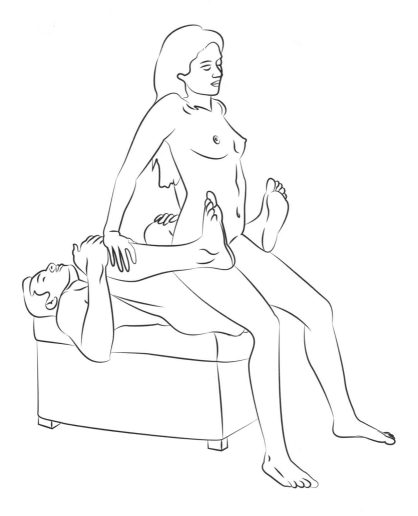

chest. She positions herself between his legs, facing out, as she lowers herself onto him. He can rest his heels on her thighs to help support her and to pull her closer.

It's a tight fit, but it gives you plenty of wiggle room to try different angles and speeds. His bent legs can help her bounce back during vigorous thrusts, and she can rock and gyrate from her perch to create deep new sensations. For bonus points, she can use one free hand to rub her clitoris while he helps support her balance by holding her other free hand or her hip.

LOVE IN BLOOM

You'll be sitting pretty with this flowery position! This move is simple to do, but the twist is in the criss-crossed legs.

He lies on the bed on his back while she climbs on top, facing his feet. She slides onto his penis, and once both partners are comfortable, she lifts and crosses her legs until she is sitting on his hips. He supports her hips with his hands to help her balance. You may have to wiggle around to get to the best position (beware of boney butts and sharp hipbones), but once

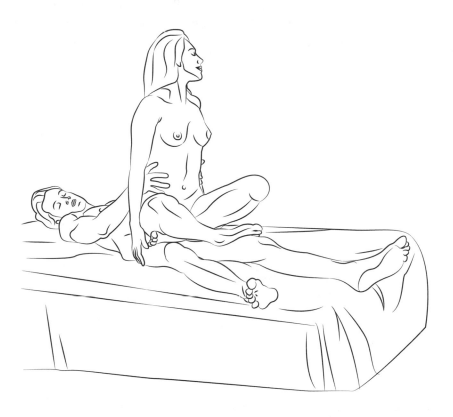

she's in place, the crossed legs give him a tighter fit, and heightens the sensations for both partners!

You won't be getting big deep thrusts with this one: she should control the action by circling and gyrating her hips while he uses his grip on her waist to pull her closer. Meanwhile she can use her free hands to rub her clitoris, or reach down between his legs to rub and fondle his balls. Or she can rest her hands on her knees and chant "OHMM!"

FRONT TO BACK

This booty-bumping position is a more sensual (and prettier!) variation on rear-entry. With your hips resting on the bed, this configuration focuses on long, slow strokes instead of fast, hard strokes with lots of motion. The result is a deliciously slow-burning ride for you both.

She lies face down, propped up on her elbows, with her legs spread. He is in the push-up position behind her, his legs on the inside of hers. As he leans forward, she arches her back, resting her head under his chin. She bends her knees to wrap her legs around his butt. If the angle's not right, putting a pillow beneath her hips will lift her pelvis for better reception. (Getting a penis through the gate is sort of crucial to sex in that

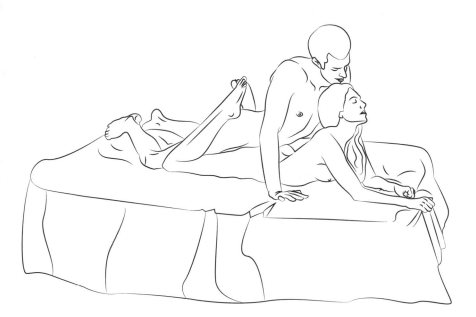

way, so it's worth being accommodating.) He may be on top, but she also has a say in the thrusting department. She can use her legs around his bum to pull him closer and meet his hips as he moves.

This position gives you lots of room for movement, so make use of it. Tilt your hips (both of you!) for a different vibe, or let your hands roam to spice up this already spicy position!

No Holds Barred

It's no secret I'm a fan of tie-'em-up games, and this position, while silver tie-free, has the perfect amount of rough stuff! Try this position when you're feeling especially naughty.

She kneels on the bed and he kneels behind her. He pushes her shoulders down on the bed while twisting her arm behind her back (Gently. If you dislocate her shoulder, YOU'RE DOING IT WRONG). He then enters her from behind. Even though she looks disarmed, she can still move her hips to meet his thrusts, or use her free hand to give herself even more traction. He can use his grip on her to help him thrust deeper. This position is begging for extras: He can add more rough to the tumble by pulling her hair or swatting her ass, and they both can break out their naughtiest dirty talk.

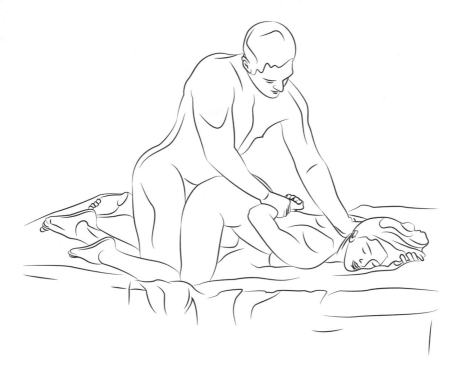

"Touch with thy lips and enkindle. This moon-white delicate body"

—Sappho, *One Hundred Lyrics*

LAID OUT

This position looks complicated, but if you take your time and move into it in steps, you'll have no trouble with it! This neat rear-entry has a feature that you often miss banging from behind: some love for the clitoris. When she bends forward, she's not just giving him a fantastic view of her ass; she's also tilting her body so that each thrust rubs her the right way.

He sits on the bed with his legs straight out in front of him. She sits on his lap with her knees outside his legs, her back against his chest, as she slides him inside of her. Once he's in position, she leans

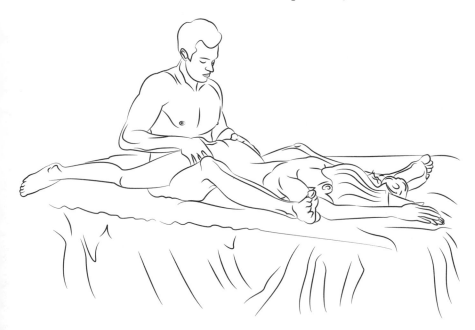

forward toward his legs as he helps tuck her legs behind him. She slowly stretches further until she is laying face down between his outstretched legs. Her hips should be up a bit, resting on his thighs, to help get the right thrusting angle. She can grab his ankles for leverage while he holds on to her hips.

RUNNING START

You'll be on the blocks constantly once you master this position. It's a hot mix of tight fit, nice view, and easy assembly, so it's a shoo-in for the gold ribbon! Try this out if you're feeling pseudo-athletic, and it will make you feel like a true Olympian!

She crouches on the bed in the runner's position, with one leg bent into a lunge and the other stretched straight back. He positions himself between her legs, straddling the outstretched leg, and kneels behind her. She supports her weight on her elbows.

Here he's got plenty of room for movement, and her back leg-front leg position makes it an extra tight squeeze. She can always switch legs if she gets tired. If she can balance it, she can use a free hand for some manual stimulation, or he can reach under her bent leg and give her a hand of his own.

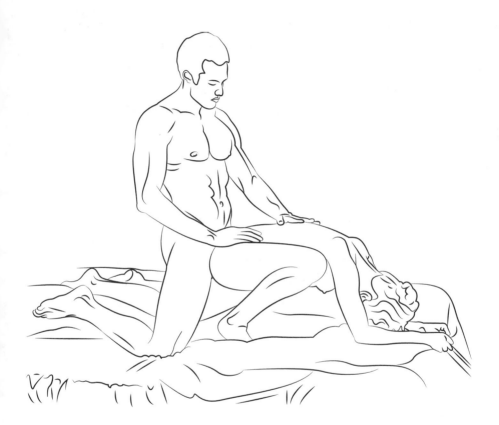

THE MERMAID

This position is a hot way to get tail—even though you need legs to make it work. You need a bit of balance to pull this move off, but it's still pretty simple (and kind of pretty!).

He sits in a big chair. She sits on his lap facing his feet and slides onto his penis. She tucks her legs behind either side of the chair as she slowly leans forward, resting her hands on his thighs. She arches her back to intensify the move.

This move is a great rear-entry position with a tight fit! The tilt of her hips gives this one a different kind of feel, and she can try leaning forward more and more to change the sensations. The more she bends, the more access he has to squeeze, smack, or fondle her ass.

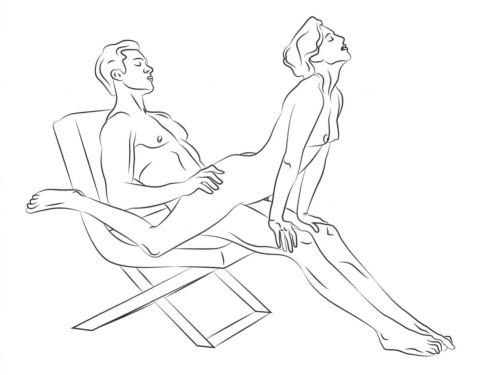

"At such a time she should take hold of her lover by the hair, and bend his head down, and kiss his lower lip, and then, being intoxicated with love, she should shut her eyes and bite him in various places."

—*The Kama Sutra*

Chapter Six

Submission

YES, PLEASE

To some, taking on the submissive role sounds like the result of a lost bet. The submissive, or "bottom," is expected to be obedient in a BDSM relationship, assuming whatever role or accepting whatever punishment his or her partner demands. Some relationships even continue this beyond the bedroom, where submissives are "slaves," or more clearly, they are consensually under the ownership of their partners, who decide various parameters of the submissives' behavior. While this kind of submission is extreme, you can explore the dynamics of submission by being held down or tied up.

When compared with the other puzzle piece, the dominant, the mere sound of being the "submissive" automatically makes it sound like it sucks. Fear not! Being the submissive is actually incredibly sexy— both because your body is chemically inclined to like it, and because in a society where upward mobility is the name of the game, lying back and taking it can feel so good. This chapter will explore why we find pleasure in a little bit of pain, and the secret no one wants you to know: being submissive actually puts you in control. If you find that you have trouble behaving, a few obedience tips will help keep you in line the next time you find yourself tied, tickled, or tamed. Do yourself a favor and submit!

THE PLEASURE OF PAIN

As a submissive, your dominant may ask you to do a full range of things during a particularly spicy tumble in bed, whether it's introducing your bare buns to an eager studded paddle, testing out those sailing knots, or taunting you with candle wax. If you've never tried any of these things out, the fear of a little bit of pain can be intimidating. Luckily, your body has natural defenses for taking these doses of discomfort and converting them into a euphoric high.

When you experience pain, whether it's stubbing your toe, cutting your finger, or getting spanked by your lover for being naughty, your brain releases endorphins, which are chemicals that connect with opiate receptors in your brain to minimize how you experience pain. They create feelings of euphoria and lower stress levels, functioning in much the same way as drugs like morphine and codeine (without the pesky drug addiction). This is where the term "runner's high," comes from; when people exercise, their brains release endorphins to distract from the exhaustion from physical activity—consider it nature's way of rewarding you for going to the gym. Certain foods are known to release endorphins as well. Unsurprisingly, chocolate is one of them—but chili peppers are, too! This is why some people love spicy foods; they know they're in for serious heat, but as they bite into that pepper and get the first bursts of spice and pain, their bodies are producing endorphins to simultaneously soothe and excite, which makes them come back for more.

Being on the receiving end of a little punishment is just like munching on chili peppers. It's spicy and a little bit nerve-racking beforehand, but your body is prepared for it. Getting spanked during a sexy session with your dominant gives your body more reasons to produce the good kind of chemicals, which can lead to an even more powerful climax.

WHAT THE DOCTOR ORDERED

The act of submission is exceptionally cathartic, relieving tension, stress, and even feelings of guilt. The average person's buildup of stress—whether from work, family, finances, or other troubles—can be overwhelming at best. Where some people choose stress reducers like cardio, yoga, or compulsively refreshing their online bank statements to make sure their bills have cleared, others go with the "fuck me and make it hurt" approach.

Relieving built-up tension is a huge part of the success of taking on the submissive role. People talk about how phenomenal makeup sex is in this way. Besides the whole, "I love you and nothing can keep us apart," aspect, this is because more often than not, you're still kind of pissed off at the person and are able to transfer your frustration into a particularly steamy and aggressive sexual romp. Makeup sex is good for the relationship, but it's also good for blowing off steam. This is how some of your submissive scenes can play out, and it's an amazing way to test your limits. There's something liberating about knowing how hard you can have your hair pulled, your lip bit, or your ass smacked during sex with your partner. Having your partner hold you down while you struggle for your reward makes that reward all the more thrilling once it's given to you.

BDSM is aggressive physical activity at its peak, which gives your body something to focus on other than whatever stress is currently weighing you down. And it's okay that this kind of intense physical activity leaves a mark. Just like getting hickeys as a teenager, physical reminders of these sessions—like a bright red handprint on your backside, or some bruising where you were tied up—are naughty little trophies for the hours or days following your sexcapades.

HOW BEING ON THE BOTTOM GIVES YOU THE UPPER HAND

In a society where compliance is a dirty word, especially for women in the workforce, being sexually submissive sounds like a kick in the shins to self-actualization and the women's movement. Not so! The reality is that in the twenty-first century, women are more and more becoming the breadwinners in their families, and represent 60% of those pursuing higher education. For both men and women, meeting goals and deadlines, buying a house, and providing for 2.5 kids and a golden retriever is all the dominance they need. Most among the hardworking task force have no greater fantasy than to just relax on a beach and do nothing—this fantasy isn't so far off from submission. Being sexually submissive allows you—whether male or female—to put aside difficult choices and the position of authority you have to assert on a daily basis. It's about being pleasured in an unconventional way by someone you trust.

Submission is sexually invigorating and therapeutic in the same way that role-playing fulfills fantasies you would otherwise not experience. In simple terms: Powerful men and women still want to be dominated. Gender roles used to insist that men be rugged, handy, and bring home the bacon, while women be sweet, feminine, and take care of the family. Now, gender roles expect that both genders do all of these things, mixing and matching, depending on the situation. Women should be powerful, pull themselves up by their bootstraps, work 40+ hours a week, and be caring wives and mothers. Men should also be powerful, pull themselves up by their bootstraps, work 40+ hours a week, and be conscientious husbands and fathers. This is an enormous amount of responsibility, considering that modern media continues to hurl conflicting expectations via cosmetic ads, airbrushed magazine covers, and reality television, ultimately confusing the shit out of you about how you're supposed to act. For these reasons, it's totally okay to want to be the business exec publicly, and slutty Susie Homemaker behind closed doors (or vice versa!). It is in no way an emasculating swat to your manhood or a degrading swipe to your female empowerment to want to be dominated.

In a submissive-dominant relationship, one of the sexiest things for the dominant is knowing that his or her submissive is conceding to certain nasty little desires in order to please. This doesn't mean that wanting to please is a one-way street, and a huge misconception about submission is that the sub has no power. True: As the bottom, you're going to be told what to do with that ice dildo and how many times to do it. False: You can't say no to the ice dildo,

"You know nothing gives me greater happiness than to serve you, to be your slave. I would give everything for the sake of feeling myself wholly in your power, even unto death."

—Leopold Sacher-Masoch
Venus in Furs

the riding crop, or the nipple clamps, and your wants don't matter. On the contrary, the submissive has the most control—perhaps not mid-throes, but definitely when lines are being drawn in the sand and limits are reached. The submissive always has veto power. Most couples make hard and soft limits very clear before going down any roads paved with floggers and chains. The sub is allowed to expressly prohibit any toys, activities, or invasions of personal boundaries. This also goes for knowing when to stop. It might be sexy as hell to count with your partner how many times he or she has smacked you with a lash-whip while you get it on, but when enough is enough, your dominant must stop when you say so. While your partner may fine-tune the details of how you receive your punishments and your rewards, as the submissive, you control the context.

OBEDIENCE TIPS

Being your dominant's naughty little girl or bad little boy requires attention to detail, endurance, and naturally, the eagerness to please. While it may be the dominant partner's job to keep the submissive in line, there are ways that the sub can harness the reins a little to fully explore his or her role as the bottom. Learning what works for you and your partner in your BDSM fantasies will improve the quality of each feisty encounter. Follow this general guide to obedience every time you find yourself stepping a toe out of line—unless, of course, you want to be punished!

SET RULES

First and foremost, you need to set rules with your dominant. Working up a 60-page contract works for some, while others are okay with sticking to scout's honor. Within these rules, you can confirm or deny the requests of your dominant, and clearly lay out how, when, and where your lusty liaisons will occur, if you so choose. Setting rules ensures that you and your partner can explore one another's curiosities without feeling uncomfortable.

HAVE A SAFEWORD

Choosing a safeword is to rough, kinky sex as landing gear is to a 747. It's really fucking important. Choose a word that is completely unrelated to the context, and one that your dominant won't mistakenly interpret as dirty talk or role-playing. Largely, words like "no," "stop," or "that hurts" can be confusing; if you're handcuffed to the bed as a high-security prisoner who needs corporal punishment, these words will only give you more of what you're getting. If you're a visual learner, elect "red" for "Stop, I've had enough," "yellow" for "Slow down or ease up," and "green" for "Hit me, baby!" If you're feeling creative, choose a family of nouns that will give the automatic signal for your partner to change what he or she is doing, whether it's "grizzly bear," "panda," and "koala" for stop, ease up, and go. If you'd rather keep it simple and use "no," or "stop," just be clear that these words have to be obeyed. Whatever you choose, make sure these words are set in stone and memorized by all.

DOMINATE YOUR SUBMISSION

Own it! Being a submissive may sound like an easy gig, but just because you're the bottom doesn't mean you get to act like a dead fish. Enthusiastically taking on your role as a sub is hard work, both physically and emotionally. Knowing this is half the battle, and the other half is doing your best to reach the goals you've set with your partner. If being the sub works for you, then revel in it! Provoke the hit from the "SLUT" paddle, tempt the cane, and invite the handcuffs. Eagerly anticipating each rough rendezvous will pay off tenfold for both you and your dom.

Chapter Seven

Domination

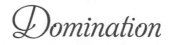

BE THE MISTER

L et out your inner dom—leather and studs optional! Playing the dom, or "top," is a challenge: You plan the games, do all of the heavy lifting, and keep a constant eye on your partner and the situation to make sure that everyone is safe, happy, and having fun. But of course, all of this work comes with some very real perks! Playing the dominant can be fun for people who already like being bossy, and it can also provide a new experience and outlet for someone who isn't used to barking orders.

Domination and submission is all about the game of power, and when you play the dom, you have all of the power. What you do with that power is up to you: You can show your partner just how much pleasure you can give him, or be selfish and command your sub to serve you. So put on (or take off?) your bossy pants and get started!

IN CHARGE

Dominance/ submission are sort of like any other sexy role-playing game you bring into your bedroom: you have to get into the spirit of the game for it to work.

What that means is up to you and your partner, since there's no "right" way to play. That doesn't mean you have to be all serious and dungeon-master-y, but you do want to feel powerful, and for your partner to feel that you're in control.

With all of the whips and chains and black leather, the dom often seems like the bad guy of the BDSM world, but that's not quite right. Remember that you aren't the villain in this scene, but the figure of authority. You're not being "mean" to your partner, you're just taking charge.

The best way to do that is to plan. The old advice is that sex should be spontaneous, spur of the moment, driven by passion. But to play dominant most effectively, you need to have a plan, if only so you can tell your partner, "Ooh baby, wait until you see what I have planned for you!"

Don't ask what your partner wants—this breaks the power dynamic you've set up, and doesn't really give your partner the submissive experience he or she is looking for. If you're just starting out, or trying something new and you're not sure how your partner will like it, you can ask "do you want me to . . . (do XYZ)," or simply tell your partner "I'm going to do this to you!" and pay attention to his response, both what he says and what his body language tells you.

THE CARE AND
KEEPING OF SUBS

Most of the focus is one-sided. The dominant partner is usually the active one, whereas the submissive is typically acted on. Everything is usually hunky-dory in BDSM land, but how can make sure it stays that way? Since you're playing with power dynamics, things can get complicated fast, and it's your responsibility as the head honcho to create a fun space for you and your partner to safely explore new feelings and push boundaries. You need to build trust with your partner—this is a new-ish kind of trust, because your sub needs to trust that you don't intend to hurt her, *and* that you are skilled enough that you know how to keep her safe. These tips can help reassure both of you on both counts. You may think that these tips will be more helpful for more advanced players, but the basics can help you and your partner avoid bruised wrists and hurt feelings, even if you're not suspending anyone from the ceiling.

Talk about it First

You probably don't need to draft a contract before you break out the blindfold, but before you try anything adventurous in bed, you're going to want to talk it over. Just as some people can't walk and chew gum at the same time, you might find it difficult to have a frank, honest talk about sex while you're actually doing it. So before you get naked, talk about it. Think about what you want and don't want during sex, go over boundaries, and be specific. If you've never really thought about this stuff before, this exercise can be enlightening.

This chat isn't a one-time discussion, either. Communication is vital to good sex, and so important to keeping BDSM play safe and fun. Check in with your partner, and ask questions when you're not sure if he or she likes what you're doing.

Once you've gone over boundaries and talked about what turns you on, you both have a much better idea of where your partner stands. The talk is just to set up guidelines, not to give one partner the green light to tie the other up and try out all of the things she didn't say "no" to.

Which brings us to . . .

Safewords

Safewords were an early kink artifact picked up by the mainstream, so most people at least know the general idea behind them. You may think that you don't need a safeword in your loving, trusting, kinky-sex-having relationship, but they can be useful for a few reasons. Having a safeword can crank up the erotic factor and help you better understand what your partner needs and wants.

The most important thing to understand about safewords is that they are not negotiable. A safeword is like an emergency ejector seat: if at any time your partner feels unsafe or uncomfortable, he or she can say the safeword, and then everything stops immediately. No one is allowed to criticize or question the use of a safeword because that is a jerk move and could make it harder for your partner to use the safeword next time she needs it. Having a safeword recognizes that your game is only happening because you both want it and are enjoying it.

As the dom, you need to make sure that your partner feels comfortable using the safeword if she needs to. But you should also be trying to make sure she never has to.

Read His Mind

An important aspect of the dom's job is empathy. You may not associate empathy with the Big Bad Dom, but BDSM works best when the top can tell what the bottom is thinking. But what if you don't have ESP? The trick is to pay attention. Watch how your partner moves, listen to his breathing, feel how he responds to you, and you'll get a pretty good idea of his mindset. Watch how he reacts when you try out different moves. If you're planning to try a new trick that neither of you has done before, take it extra slow. If possible, you should try things out yourself before you inflict them on your partner. For example, if you're going to be using hot wax, test out how the wax feels on your own body before you go dripping it all over your partner. You can see how this can help you keep your games safe and fun— you're less likely to accidentally burn your partner if you know what you're working with!

You Make the Rules

Now that you're versed in the responsibilities, it's time to get you cracking the (figurative) whip! One of the best ways to flex your authority is by issuing orders and setting rules. If your partner fails to follow directions, you get to decide what punishment to hand out. These commands and rules don't have to be all about sex—you're showing your partner that you're in charge, so your orders should emphasize that you're the boss. Your rules should be arbitrary—that's the point! The rules are only there so that you can enforce them, and so that your partner can submit to them.

Just as with everything else in this book, there's no right or wrong way to do this. There's a huge range of ways that people act out this power play, and you don't have to wear a leash and call each other "slave" and "master" (unless you want to). Getting into your roles can be an adjustment, so take it slow like with the other moves. Here are some ideas to get you started:

Say my Name

Have your partner call you something sexy. You could go with the basic "Sir," or "Ma'am," or even "Master," but if that feels more silly than sexy, come up with something on your own. Submissives often refer to themselves in third person, which can get tricky if you're not used to it, so that might be a fun challenge to add to your play.

Fetch

Order your partner to get something for you. Whatever you want: a glass of water, a magazine, or that toy from across the room. You can think of this as a standard "because I said so" kind of command—whatever the exact reason for of the request, the real purpose is just to exercise your power.

Playing Dress Up

Tell your sub what to wear. This is fun just for sexy time, especially if you have some sexy lingerie or kinky costumes to bust out. Or have your partner wear something sexy just for you before they head out for the day: it could be their sexiest underoos, or some special jewelry or accessory.

Punishment

You've laid down the law, but it doesn't mean anything without a little enforcement. In fact, it is much better to think of your role as the dom to be enforcing, rather than punishing. When you're playing BDSM and your partner breaks a rule or disobeys orders, a "punishment" is useful to reinforce the dom's authority and the rules of the game. It can also give you a good chance to try some spanking techniques that you both enjoy in a "realistic" context.

Think about your punishment like the penalty in a drinking game. It's like when you miss a shot in beer pong and you have to chug—it's not personal, and it's not because the dom is angry with the sub for breaking the rules; it's just how you play the game. With that in mind, you should also remember that BDSM is *not* the time to work through real-life conflicts, and you should never punish your partner for real-world transgressions.

How you hand out your punishments, and what kind of punishments you use is entirely up to you, so be creative! Your punishments don't have to be painful—in fact, unless you both enjoy a little pain with your pleasure, you can leave the belt at the door.

When you're playing around in the bedroom, it can be fun to issue sexy orders. You can have your partner touch themselves, or do something for you. You might want to think twice before choosing a sexytime staple as your punishment—do you really want to characterize a blow job as "punishment?" So make your "punishment" something new—you have a whole book of ideas here to choose from.

To really flex your dom muscles, you can assign punishments that benefit you—you are the boss, after all. Have your sub rub your feet, fix you a drink, maybe braid your hair or do your laundry. Think outside the box on this one.

You can even make a punishment game with your partner by making a list of possible punishments beforehand, and numbering the list. Then when you need to punish your partner, have them roll a set of dice. Whatever number they land on is the punishment you use. If you don't have dice, you can write them on slips of paper and draw them from a hat. This works well if you two switch roles.

IT'S YOUR SCENE

In the kink world these pre-planned sexcapades are called "scenes." That term works so well because even if you're not wearing a costume, you are putting on a show. The end game is for you and your partner

"Oh then! the fiery touch of his fingers determines me, and my fears melting away before the glowing intolerable heat, my thighs disclose of themselves, and yield all liberty to his hand."

—John Cleland
Fanny Hill: or, the Memoirs of a Woman of Pleasure

to have a good time, and the dom gets to make sure that happens—you're the director. For this you have to plan ahead. What kinds of props do you want to use? What toys or accessories? Are you going to tie your partner up or leave 'em loose? You can mix and match the moves in this book, and add in your own flourishes as you go.

When you put on a scene, you get to control all the little details, and as you play with bondage, submission, and sensations, you get to control what your partner feels and experiences. How delicious— absolute power! Your partner's tied to the tracks, and what part will you play? Are you the dastardly villain, the courageous hero . . . or are you the train?

When preparing for a scene, think about how your partner will experience everything you have planned. Even if you're just planning a simple bedroom romp, you can help your sub get into the groove by making sure the room temperature is comfortable, clearing any clutter that could get in your way, and removing things that could distract your sub, like pictures, the alarm clock, or anything like that. Think through the whole plan, and make sure you have everything you need. When you're finally ready for your sub, suit up and get ready to put on a show.

Chapter Eight

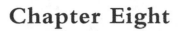

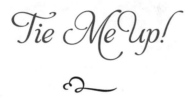

"Thou art to me a **delicious torment.**"

—Ralph Waldo Emerson

"Cupid kills with arrows, some with traps."

—Shakespeare
Much Ado about Nothing

WHY TIE?

P laying with ropes with your partner takes a lot of trust, but that can make it even sexier! Part of the fun of bondage is the sense of adventure with a touch of role play. Trussed up and helpless, you get to play the damsel in distress, or tie the ropes yourself to play the villain!

The most important element of bondage is the perception of control. Your knots do not have to be flawless; you're not rigging a sailboat, and your partner is not going to drift away on the tide. But you should bind your partner so that it feels real; like good theater, to get the best effect everyone has to play along, but it would be hard to get into the story if the actors had cardboard swords, and you'll feel silly thrashing sexily against uselessly loose bindings. So pick your props with an eye for style, and stick to the scene!

Let's get serious for a second. Sex is awesome, but sex-related accidents are less so. So don't be dumb: think ahead, and never leave a person tied up alone. Always have a way to free your partner quickly, in case of fire, flood, or zombie apocalypse. Only play tie-up games with partners you trust to untie you, and always respect your partner's boundaries.

Look, No Hands!

cͻ⁓

Tying your partner up isn't just supposed to keep him or her still; by binding your partner's wrists, you take away the freedom to use hands for anything at all! Restraining your partner's hands sends a powerful message that you are in control and in charge of what's happening. This message is as visual and symbolic as it is "real," so even with this simple move you have a thousand ways to make it yours.

Sitting, standing, bent over the couch or propped against the back of an elevator—you can play this game anywhere; the only rule is that for one of you, it's hands-off! Think of this as bondage practice, or the smallest unit of bondage. Simply, one partner loses the use of their hands. You can do this in many ways: while riding on top, hold your partner's hands down with your own, or order your partner to keep the hands above the head on threat of punishment. Of course, for the true bondage feel, you need some kind of physical binding—a tie, perhaps?

You can tie wrists together with hands positioned palm to palm, or have the wrists crossed. With palms together, the bound partner can move around and readjust if the bindings become uncomfortable, but some prefer the more elegant look of the crossed wrists. Depending on what activities you have in mind, you can decide to bind hands in front or behind the back. Having your hands bound behind your back can be more challenging than having them tied in front: It affects your balance and makes you more susceptible to falling, all of which also makes you feel more vulnerable (and makes you stick your chest out a bit, which your partner may enjoy as an extra perk!). If you're going to be moving around, it may be easier to keep hands tied in front; that way you are free to help with blow job positioning and flicking hair out of your eyes, but not so free that you have any control. That feeling of helplessness is the flip side of the powerful feeling you get when you tie your partner up, but like we found out with spanking, the partner on top isn't the only one enjoying the game!

Tied Up and Teased

It's all well and good to say you're going to tie your partner up, but then what? You want to change things up, not just have the same sex you always have with a few extra accessories. You want to make the most of your situation, and the best way to do that is with some well-placed caresses. The goal is twofold: you want to drive your partner crazy with soft strokes that almost—but not quite!—send them off, and you want to flaunt your powerful position by taking your time and putting your hands all over your playmate.

For this you only need a partner and something to tie him up with. There are plenty of things you can find around the house for this purpose: scarves, belts, and ties work well, especially to start, as do things like stretchy fabric bandages, fuzzy handcuffs, and so on! Start small until you know what you and your partner are comfortable with. If you decide to use something that fastens or ties securely, like plastic zip ties, rope or cord, make sure you have scissors nearby in case you have to remove the bindings quickly. Wrists and ankles are the parts you'll most likely want to secure, but use caution, since both areas are chock-full of sensitive nerves, tendons, and arteries. Don't let your bindings cut off circulation, and if you're going to put any pressure or weight on the bindings, you should spread out the weight by tying multiple points along the same limb. If you're planning to get extra-freaky, you can also buy cuffs and bindings made especially for bondage play, and with safety and style in mind. These come in a variety of materials and types of fastenings. Keep the bindings snug but with a bit of give, so that your partner is comfortable and can wiggle around a little. Your partner might also like to have the bindings positioned so that he has a hand-hold—something to grip in the throes of passion.

Once your partner is securely bound, don't rush to the erogenous zones; instead, touch and kiss your partner slowly along the sternum, all the way down to the abs. This area is very sensitive in its own right, and it has prime real estate right by your partner's naughty bits. Spend some time here, but don't be tempted to move further south: you want to delay gratification for you and your partner, so don't head straight for home plate (or third base . . . listen, forget sports, just don't let anybody come yet). You can tease with gentle strokes or "accidental" grazes against your partner's sexy parts, but don't linger in any one spot too long. Move slowly, and emphasize your control over the situation by touching your partner in unpredictable patterns and drawing out the foreplay. Remember, this isn't just an excuse to feel your partner up unhindered (although you can certainly do that too): touch him the way you know he likes it, and if you're not sure where that is, then this is the time to find out! After a bit more teasing, you can take pity on your partner and start dealing out that gratification you've been delaying! Like before, don't spend too long in any one place, but switch up your moves as soon as your partner seems to get used to what you're doing. Once your partner is writhing and ready, you can choose how to finish him off, with a tantalizing blow job, a fast and furious cowgirl romp, or however you'd like—it's up to you!

BOUND AND RUBBED DOWN

Massages are a classic sexytime move found in even the most vanilla of bedrooms. Rub-downs are hot: the feel of skin on skin, soft moans of pleasure, the physicality of the whole process—all of it is a steamy way to ramp up your tryst. When you add a little bondage to the mix, the combination can be explosive! Just like with the "tie up and tease" move, this trick is all about control. You are in control of your partner's body, and lucky for him or her, you're planning to be nice—for now! You can get a thrill manhandling your helpless partner, and being a bit pushy with your kneading, but the real fun is seeing how many ways you can make your partner beg for more!

By now you should be a pro at tying your partner up. For this move, it's especially important to keep the bindings loose and comfortable; you want him to pay attention to what you're doing, not be distracted by the rope cutting into his wrist. You can tie your partner lying face-up to start, or find a comfortable way to bind him so you have full access to his back end.

You can set the scene with solid old-school tricks, like lowering the lights, putting on some soft music, and lighting some candles to add needed ambience. Massage oil adds a nice touch as well, or you can use a nice-smelling lotion. And remember that massage oil works on more places than just the back!

To begin, warm up your hands, with or without massage oil, and then gently place your hands on your partner. Pause there for a moment, and then start your massage. Start by kissing your partner, and work your hands behind his head. As you're kissing, gently press your fingers along your partner's spine, starting at the base of his skull. This spot is filled with sensitive nerve endings and pressure points; combined with your kissing, this gentle touch will get you both in the right mindset. Don't spend too much time there, because although it feels heavenly, too much rubbing there can give your partner a headache or leave him sore. As you move further south, concentrate on the bigger muscles like in the arms and shoulders. Make sure to alternate between strong rubbing on the bigger areas and gentle touching on other sensitive places like wrists, hands, and feet. You can get a bit rough (since you're in charge) but be careful not to hurt your partner; a pushy rubdown is hot, a sore muscle or a pinched nerve is not. Pay attention to the noises your partner is making. You know the sounds your partner makes when he's feeling good, so listen for the tell-tale sighs or moans that say you've hit the right spot. You can keep your massage going for as long as you want, then you can decide to end your game by finishing your partner off with your hands, your mouth, or by riding him home.

Using Restraint: Tied Down

There are plenty of ways to tie up your partner, but you can't beat the tried-and-true spread-eagle position. It's a comfortable position that doesn't require any strange body contortions, but leaves the bound partner accessible and at your mercy. Lots of the fun of this move comes from the look of the position itself. The perfect picture of the effect of this move can be intense because your hands and feet are bound, but that only makes the end result even more explosive!

This move is easy for anyone with a big bed with head and footboards, but if your sex cave is still under construction, you can make a few changes to get any bedroom a-rocking. You can buy cheap drawer handles, or even just a few eye hooks, and secure them to your bed frame or the wall behind your bed, in suitable "spread-eagle" placements. You may not want to do this if you're afraid of being found out, but the small hooks shouldn't be too noticeable depending on where you install them. For a much more subtle option, you can invest in a set of specially-made bondage sheets with anchors for straps built right in, or you can get a similar effect by running some rope or bungee cord underneath your mattress. Get creative and you should be able to find a good solution for your situation.

Whether by hook or by headboard, your next step is to tie 'em down. Each hand is tied separately to the bed or hook, and the ankles are secured with the legs spread apart. If you're being tied up, make sure you're comfortable, because you'll be here a while! With this move the bound partner has even less physical control over the situation, which can be seriously heady! Remember, even though you are tied down, you can help control the action with verbal cues. This is especially fun and helpful as you're starting out, because you have to think about and put into words what you want and where you want it. Once you get more comfortable you can change the rules, and let your partner find his own way to drive you crazy.

PLAYING ALONG: TIED SITTING

Sex tied to the bed is exciting, but it's still . . . sex in a bed. There are plenty of other pieces of furniture around your house that you can use to strap in! Chairs are great and give you a different experience from being tied to the bed—the restrained partner is sitting up and can look around while still being securely tied up.

There are a few ways to tie someone to a chair, and they mostly depend on what chair you have in mind. Kitchen chairs usually have plenty of slats and dowels to tie things to, and are made of solid wood or other materials that are easy to clean after the fun. If your chair has arms, they make good places to secure the bound partner's wrists, but this configuration can limit access and movement more than you'd like. With an armless chair, you can have your wrists tied behind your back or secured to the sides of the chair. Securing the feet is easy: Ankles can be tied to the chair legs or each other, with the knees pushed together or pulled wide, depending on what you have planned! When playing around with bondage and smaller furniture like chairs, make sure that the chair is on a solid surface and watch that it doesn't fall over during your sexcapade.

Since the sitting position gives your partner a good view, use this to your advantage and put on a show. You have an audience, so enjoy it. You can put on a sexy lap dance or striptease, or don a costume or sexy accessories and enjoy the fact that your partner can only look, not touch! Unlike earlier moves where you wanted your touches to be surprising and unexpected, here you want to telegraph your touches, to let your partner know "I'm going to touch you here . . . because I said so!"

The downside of the chair position is that it limits access to most of the sexy bits, especially if the bound partner is of the vagina-having variety. You can get around this by relegating the chair to foreplay, and activating your ejector button (or just untying the knots) before you both finish, or you can go the distance by getting creative and a little flexible. If your partner is a guy, your job's a bit easier. You can give

The only way to
get rid of a
temptation
is to
yield to it."

—Oscar Wilde
The Picture of
Dorian Gray

him a toe-curling blow job, and he's got a front-row seat. If your chair is sturdy, you can climb on board and enjoy some hot face-to-face chair sex.

ON YOUR KNEES

Bondage is about power and control, so what better way to show that than with some bondage keeping you on your knees? Kneeling is a powerful symbol of submission, so this move will be extra-thrilling for the bound partner, who gets to play at being helpless and dominated, and for the dominating partner, who enjoys this display of subservience from a higher, more powerful position.

There are many ways to bind your partner kneeling. You don't have to do a full-body binding—you can use the techniques discussed earlier to bind your partner's wrists, commanding them to kneel, or guiding/physically positioning them with your hands. This kind of external power play can be extra sexy paired with the submissive position. If you want the full bondage solution, you can try a variation on the Hog Tie position, which I'll talk more about later. For this move, have the bound partner kneel in a comfortable position, with hands at his or her sides. Then tie each wrist to the corresponding ankle (left to left, etc.), leaving enough rope so that the bound partner can still kneel comfortably, but not so loose that they can use their hands. This position can make the bound partner lose balance, and with the hands bound, he or she won't be able to stop a fall, so keep a supportive hand on your partner, and never leave him or her alone.

The kneeling position is nice to look at, and it puts the bound partner at just about the perfect height to perform some oral sex. If you have trouble making that work comfortably with the bound partner kneeling and the other standing, try using different chairs or sitting on the edge of the bed. However you make it work, this move hits you with a double-whammy of hot visuals and good positioning.

FANCY ROPE WORK

If ropes have gotten your motor running, you're in luck! There's an almost endless number of ways to tie someone up, as long as you have enough rope and a willing partner. Different bondage configurations work for different kinds of games and positions. In all cases, the fun is in the power play, but also partly in the theater of the game. Advanced bondage steps up the intensity on both fronts: With these tricks the partner on top has more control, and the partner set to be tied has even less, and less chance of movement, as well. Advanced rope work often also looks cooler, and more intense, which multiplies the effect. These tricks come with the same warnings as before: Be smart, use common sense, and don't ever leave your partner tied up alone. Because these tricks involve more rope covering more of your body, they can be a tad more dangerous than beginner moves. But when you're playing safely, these ramped-up moves can make your sex sesh incredibly kinky and fun!

Hog Tie:

You've probably heard the term "hog tied" before, since it's a pretty common term that people use to simply mean "tied up completely." In this case, hog tying is a specific rope arrangement where the person's wrists and ankles are fastened and drawn together with another binding, either in front or behind the back. This position makes it impossible for the bound partner to move. First, bind your partner's wrists together, then the ankles. Then grab another rope and run it through (or otherwise connect it to) the bindings around the wrists and ankles. Adjust the connector rope to pull the wrists and ankles closer together, only as much as is comfortable. Now review your work—you have a neatly-tied gift laid out in front of you! You may not actually be able to have sex with your partner in this position, but it works great for foreplay, or for dom/sub role-play.

Frogtie:

The frogtie is a more utilitarian version of the hog tie that gives you access to the bound partner's sexy bits, allowing you to use this position during oral sex, while playing with toys, and a whole bunch of other fun activities. There are variations to this move. The more advanced technique involves tying one's ankles to the calves, right at the hip, so that the knees are kept bent (like a frog's, apparently) and the bound person is unable to move. The simpler way to accomplish this move is to fasten each wrist to the corresponding ankle. This gives the bound partner more wiggle room than the trickier version, but it's also more comfortable and easier to accomplish. This technique is great because it works for a bunch of different positions. The bound partner can lie down, with her arms by her side, which pulls her ankles back and apart, or she can sit up or be propped up against a headboard.

A more grueling version of this is the Leapfrog position. Essentially this is the frogtie with the bound partner lying face down. It can become painful quickly, so don't plan to spend too much time in this position, since it puts so much strain on the neck and shoulders. To accomplish this position, have the bound partner kneel on the bed, (if you're doing this somewhere other than the bedroom, make sure the surface you're on is soft and comfortable, or this will hurt!). Pull each arm down and between the legs, and fasten it to the corresponding ankle (right to right, etc.). When that's done, the bound partner will be lying with her head and shoulders pressed against the bed, with her ass in the air. This is a hot position for spanking or rear-entry, and it just plain looks sexy!

The Ball Tie:

This position is so simple and easy to do, and works with so many different sex positions, that it's a wonder that it hasn't gained more notoriety. Lie back on the bed, then pull your knees up to your chest, like you're curling up into a ball. Wrap your arms around your legs, and have your partner secure your wrists together. Voilà! With one small binding you are now an incapacitated ball of sex, you sexy thing, you! This position leaves your ass and sexy bits exposed, making this trick perfect for pre-spanking bondage.

MORE BINDING OPTIONS

Now that I've shown you the ropes, feel free to get creative with some other exciting bondage equipment. That old tie you've been using is getting a bit ratty. . . .

Leather

Leather bindings are both comfortable and sturdy, with a nice sheen and a look that means business. Accessories can make a big difference in bondage play, since it helps you get into the spirit of the game, so bringing leather into your bed can be extra kinky!

Basic leather gear includes leather cuffs, collars, and other more mainstream sexy garments like bustiers and corsets. These can be useful in bondage play, since they often have straps that make them easy to fasten to other things. The real perk of leather accessories is the look: leather is just sexy. And since it's the look you want, if you or your partner is vegan you can find all sorts of classy faux-leather online.

Metal

Metal bonds are useful because they are strong, sturdy, and tend to be latched or fastened in a way that makes them easy to put on and remove quickly. Metal bindings like handcuffs can be less comfortable than softer bindings, and they may leave marks if the bound partner pulls against them, so keep that in mind when you plan your scenes.

Metal bindings are fairly basic. You have the typical wrist cuffs and ankle cuffs, along with the more exotic thumb cuffs. You can also find "fuzzy" cuffs, which are lined with some other material to make them more comfortable. For more advanced play, you can find bars and spreaders to hold apart the bound partner's ankles, or to bind their arms, like stocks. Metal, like leather, is used for its looks: metal bindings are hard, cold, and unyielding, making this material well suited for a rougher tumble.

Rope

There are a ton of different kinds of rope you can use for bondage play, and there are even more kinds of rope that are *not* for bondage. You can find rope at most home improvement stores (if you have to ask, just say you're building a tire swing or something—you may want to leave this book at home). Find a rope that's soft on your skin, and that can hold a knot. Materials like cotton, nylon, or hemp are a good bet. If you're looking for something rougher, look for sisal rope or some other natural fiber. While you're at the store, you may want to look for eye hooks or anchors you can attach to your bed to make for some fun rope configurations.

Other Stuff

If you really want to play with bondage, you can get almost anything you need from a sex store online. Yeah, you can play with stuff you have, but the best accessories are the ones that were made for the job. Two great tools you can get are velcro straps and bondage tape.

Velcro straps are quick to secure, like leather or metal cuffs, but they're a whole lot more comfortable. With straps, you can try out positions that were too difficult to tie on your own. You can get wrist and ankle straps, which work like cuffs, or straps designed for a specific position, like hog tie straps.

Bondage tape is great, and it's the only kind of tape you should ever use for bondage, because it's specially made to be put on skin. Other types of tape, especially something strong like duct tape, can be difficult to remove safely; bondage tape, though, can be used as a binding, as a blindfold, or almost anything you want.

Chapter Nine

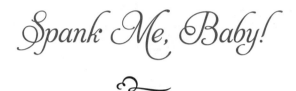

Spank Me, Baby!

"Pain is no evil,
Unless it
conquers us."

—Charles Kingsley

"Sweet is pleasure
after pain."

—John Dryden
Alexander's Feast

THE HOWS AND WHYS
OF SPANKING

⌒2⌒

Before there were sex playrooms, before there were dildos, and before there were floggers, even, there was an open palm. Spanking is the very first step into the painfully hot side of your sexy rendezvous, with a little something for everyone. While there's no question why the sweet sides of sex keep hot-blooded bodies coming back for more, it's harder to imagine why a good wallop would have the same effect. As it turns out, your body releases chemicals, like endorphins and adrenaline, when triggered by strenuous activity, stimulation, and even pain—a trifecta that is abundant during sex. So when your partner's brimming lust gets hand-delivered, the combination of your arousal and a little surge of pain can bring your romp, and eventual climax, to a whole new level. Beginning with baby steps (or maybe baby spanks!) this chapter will show you the A-Zs of one of the most exciting and simple additions to your sexual repertoire.

THE BAREHANDED BENCHMARK

If you have never felt the tingle of a freshly spanked rump, it's best to start with the basics. No, not the flogger; we'll get there. First, start with what you were born with: your bare hands. Whether you want to be the spanker or the spankee, barehanded spanking is a way to tap into a lusty—even primal—side of sex. It can also be an amazing way to connect with your partner mid-romp. While spanking can involve games of power play, in the throes of sex spanking is more often than not, a reaction—as our team of scientists like to call it, the "OMG, you feel amazing. I just have to grab or hit something!" response. Whichever your fancy, doing it barehanded will inspire a new side of your sex life that is stingingly sweet. So warm up those palms or scoot up your bum, and let the spanking begin!

With the beginning stages of spanking, you have to test the waters before you jump in. As the spanker, if you're unsure if your partner wants to try spanking with you, and you fear "the Talk" try warming up with it the next time she's on top. Caress or massage her ass a little, and when you're feeling particularly enthralled, give her a swift—but not too swift—smack to the bum. Body language (or her screaming your name) should indicate whether you have the green light or a halting red stop sign.

Once you have the go-ahead, treat spanking like candy. If you have too little, you might be missing out on something sweet. If you have too much, you've spoiled an appetite and you might never be allowed back in the candy store again. Incorporate palm-to-cheek meetings when things are particularly fiery to send both of your sexual trajectories soaring. Feel free to spank multiple times in a row with a slow, firm rhythm, either open-palmed or with your palm slightly cupped. This can occur with the spankee on top ("The Reach Around," if you will), or doggie-style, where you'll have a better view of the bright red handprint you'll be making on your partner's tush.

The subtle nuances of asking to be spanked aren't much different than asking to spank. If you and your partner have good sexual chemistry, chances are that the risk of asking is worth the reward. Declaring, "I want you to spank me," while out to dinner with the in-laws may not be the right way to go about it, but kissing your partner's neck and whispering it in his ear while you're on top of him in bed just might. If you're uncomfortable with asking directly, move your partner's hands to your hips during sex, and slowly bring them to cup or squeeze your ass. Go so

"No empty-handed
man can lure
a bird."

—Geoffrey Chaucer
The Canterbury Tales

far as to take your partner's hands and do the smack-
ing yourself. At that point, he or she should be able
to infer that you're saying, "Spank me, baby!"

PROPPING IT UP

After you and your partner have covered the basics
of barehanded, it's time to use a prop. Using a prop
while spanking will increase your ability to deliver
a good thump, or intensify a spanking that you're
about to receive. With every good thwap to the ass
you enjoy, more blood flows to the very sensitive
nerve endings in the cheeks, which also means more
blood flow and impact are sent to the very sensitive
nerve endings located right next door. Incorporating
props is an exciting way to liven up your sex life, not
just because it's something new, but also because it
involves forethought. While spontaneous sex is nothing to scoff at, there's something undeniably sexy
about knowing your partner thinks about doing you
so often that he or she went out and bought a toy.

The props you and your partner use don't necessarily need to have blockbuster production value.
You can use household items like the time-honored

classics, the hairbrush and the ping-pong paddle. Both of these items are easily wielded, and while they'll certainly pack some punch, the spankee won't necessarily fear sitting down for the next week. A ping-pong paddle is usually encased in a thin layer of leather or rubber, which will end each blow with a slick smack. A hairbrush is more multifaceted. The flat end of the brush will deliver much the same impact as the paddle, while the bristled end (either hair or plastic with soft nubs) will add a prickly sensation to switch up the feel of each cheeky encounter.

If you're looking for an excuse to buy your props, there are paddles available that will bring your spanking session anywhere from sweetly sensual all the way to nastily naughty. For the former effect, try using a fur-lined paddle. The fuzzy addition to a firm paddle softens the sting of spanking, and can also be used to massage, caress, and seduce the spankee throughout its use. If you'd prefer something with ten times the zing, studded paddles are the take-no-prisoners approach to dishing out a good thumping. The studs create further pressure points to spike up the sexy mix of pleasure and pain. With these tools under your belt (you can use that, too!), your armory of sexilicious spankers is well on its way!

Teach Me a Lesson

An armory of spanking techniques must be accompanied by a bit of role-playing. Whether you're dressing up as a leather-clad dominatrix, a sexy cop, a dirty doctor, or a naughty [insert profession here], role-playing gives an adrenaline shot to your sexcapades. The key to these games, of course, is doing the things you wouldn't do in everyday life, particularly if it has a pinch of spice and feels a little bit wrong. Sure, you might not normally go hiking, but role-playing as two adoring lovers in a mountainside field of lilacs isn't what you're looking for to sexify your lust sessions (unless it involves ropes and carabiners). So be the bad girl or the naughty boy and go for the Oscar in your next performance.

For simplicity's sake, let's pretend you and your partner want to live out the Naughty Schoolgirl fantasy. It may sound overdone, but there's a reason why Britney Spears's "Baby One More Time" was so damn successful: It's hot. Not only is it super sexy, but it's a low-maintenance and low-cost way to get your and your partner's blood pumping.

First, pick out the wardrobe. Shopping online for schoolgirl skirts is a sure thing; otherwise, try second-hand, or of course, your local naughty gift shop. Once you have your costume, you're nearly ready for that after school special. Pair the skirt with whichever tightly fitting button-up blouse, T-shirt, or cardigan you already own, a pair of knee socks, and high heels—preferably Mary Janes, if you have them. Add some pigtails or French braids, and you've got one sexy schoolgirl on your hands.

Staying in character is one of the more important challenges of role-playing. Saying, "this is stupid," and "I feel silly," with stiff body language is the fastest way to get a big fat F on your exam. Confidence is sexy, so take control of your end of the bargain, whether it's the naughty schoolgirl or the professor she's staying after class with. Use your Dirty Talk Do's to get the scene playing out: Bite your lip as you tell your "professor" how badly you need to practice for your oral exams, or give your schoolgirl some corporal punishment for not handing in her homework on time. Making varsity never felt so good!

No schoolgirl scenario—or role-playing scenario, for that matter—would be complete without a nice dose of spanking. The point is to be bad, so get your palms, ruler, or clipboard out to give some serious detention. Bend your schoolgirl over your knee to punish her for being too cheeky, asking her to count as you spank and call you sir. Schoolgirl skirts are short for a reason, so make good use of them! Pull her skirt up and use your thick dictionary to remind her why she's staying after class. Those pigtails aren't just for show, either. Whether you're the one pulling her hair or getting your hair pulled, a little animalistic aggression will get you everywhere in your dirty scene. Pigtails are a perfect hairdo for a from-behind ride, so pull her by the reins and slap her ass to get her really going.

Step up your sexy performance: buy additional props for spanking and branch out to different roles, even if it means that she's the whistling construction worker and he's the innocent passerby. Have fun with your wicked side and break the rules!

TOYS YOUR PARENTS NEVER GAVE YOU

For the ever-curious, here is a list of toys that will get you itching for a good spanking!

Feather Tickler: A sultry and seductive way to begin with naughty play, a feather tickler is a sexy, more colorful (and cleaner) version of the French maid variety feather duster. Use it to taunt and tease your partner until he or she is writhing for you!

Riding Crop: Like the ones brandished at the Kentucky Derby, a riding crop is a standard tool for BDSM play. A long rod with a gripping handle, the tip has a small leather fold that will really get your attention on contact.

Plastic or Wooden Cane: Best used for corporal punishment for your lover, a cane is usually lightweight and flexible—it's a tool you can hear coming.

Paddles: There are dozens of different kinds of paddles, which are long, flat pieces of wood (sometimes bound in vinyl or leather) or plastic with short handles. Fur lined paddles give a softer blow; studded paddles pack prickly heat; paddles with holes will bring your swing down with a serious whip; and impression paddles leave marks ranging from cutesy hearts to words like "LOVE" or "SLUT."

Cat o' Nine Tails: A type of flogger, cat o' nine tails have a gripping rod with long leather tails for that feline lashing.

Lash Whip: In the flogging category as well, a lashing whip has a leather handle, often with braided tails that are knotted at the end, with smaller tails stemming from the knots. This whip is for serious BDSM play.

Spanking Gloves: To keep the contact coming, leather spanking gloves will protect your hands from the zing of barehanded blows and boost the impact for your partner. Some gloves are lined with stippling to further exaggerate the sting.

Leather Spanking Skirt: For the spanking seductress, these soft leather skirts are tailored to look like sexy, knee-length pencil skirts from the front, but leave the wearer bare-bottomed in the back for optimal access. Leather straps keep the skirt in place and create a hot bondage look.

"Would you do me
the great kindness,
Madame,
of allowing me to bite
and pinch your
lovely flesh while
I'm at my fuckery?"

—Marquis de Sade
Philosophy in the Bedroom

Flog Me Gently

⌒⌒

Flogging takes prop use to the next level (or five). A typical flogger is a spanking device that has a handle (otherwise known as a "pommel") with flowing tails attached, generally of the same length. These tails can be made up of leather, rubber, plastic, rope, horse hair, chain, or other materials, and can be used in a variety of ways throughout your mischievous spanking session. Floggers can be used to discipline your naughty partner, or to push your limits further than you ever thought you could go and then some. This kind of erotic play is the ultimate destination for endorphin junkies. The more pain you take from your partner's flogger, the more you gain from that sweet release. From punishment and dominance play to flogging on a whim, this method of nasty pleasure makes even Catwoman purr.

The flogger is most often used for "discipline" purposes, where the spankee lies face down or leans over a chair, table, pillow, or even your very own spanking bench. The flogger can be administered with rapid flicks, which will bite steadily at the skin to get you and your partner hollering with excitement. For more sting to your swing, use a harder, slower pace, which will deliver a serious smack, as well as heighten anticipation between each impact. Before, after, or in between, lightly drag the tails of the flogger along your partner's ass or future flog-zone to tickle and taunt. This will provide relief in between blows, as well as get your partner all tingly with goose bumps for the next round.

Knowing which regions to target is extremely important. Generally speaking, the areas that scream "flog me!" are the back of the thighs, the shoulders, and of course, that booty. Unless you and your partner think a stint in the emergency room or a jail cell is super hot, it is important to stay away from the head, face, neck, spine, and soft tissue like the stomach, where all those important organs hang out. Flogging can be ultra sexy, but it's important to use your toys safely!

Pardon the yuck, but keep your flogger clean! Flogging isn't for the faint of . . . well, the faint . . . so if your sessions are especially intense, be prepared for welts and even broken skin or bleeding. Never use an unwashed flogger for multiple partners, and when you do clean it after each use, use disinfectants like antibacterial soap, leather cleaner, and bleach, depending on the material of the flogger. When you have these bases covered, flog it out of the park!

THE POST-SPANKING POSTERIOR

With every good spanking, there needs to be equally good aftercare. Spanking play is to test your physical limits and invigorate your sexuality, to find new ways to bond with your partner, and naturally, to arouse. The best spanking rendezvous shouldn't leave you or your partner trembling in a corner after you've finished. If you are setting out for a no-holds-barred approach to spanking and BDSM play, then the post-spanking massage is a must-do to come down from a painfully good spanking summit and soothe those rosy cheeks.

There's no doubt about it—spanking is an ass kicking. Whether the red-hot mark left on you or your partner's glutes is in the shape of a hand that meant business, the tip of a riding crop, or reads the word "SLUT" from a particularly naughty paddle you purchased, they're going to need some attention. Lay the spankee down on the bed, your lap, or another soft surface, and lightly caress along the back, then the thighs, and then slowly begin to massage the bare bum. If you still feel like role-playing, tell the spankee he or she has done a good job and deserves the massage being given—anything negative is a Dirty Talk Don't. Rub massage oils or calming creams on areas that were given the most attention during the spanking. If you suspect there will be bruising (or can already see it), the massage will reduce soreness and increase circulation. Aftercare isn't just about the physical strain of spanking, it's also emotionally important. If your spanking exploits are particularly rough, the spankee may need a little extra affection and reminders of self-worth. Any games of power play and possibly degradation need to be cut as soon you've finished so there is no emotional confusion.

When choosing massage oils and creams, it is important to know what you're looking for. If you want to go all natural, essential oils like eucalyptus will be a wakeup for the skin, whereas jasmine and lavender will be more calming. If purchased in pure form, these oils *need* to be diluted with other base oils like almond or sesame, because large doses can be toxic and even lethal (read the labels!!!). To skip the worry, just buy scented massage oils in your local bath shops. Choose scents that won't overwhelm, and avoid oils and creams that contain alcohol, because they'll sting—and not in a sexy way. Some of the best rubdown elixirs are those with aloe vera, shea butter, vitamin E, and warming massage oils. The warming sensation will soothe the skin and help both you and your partner relax after all that hard work. With any luck, your massage will be so soothing and sensual that you might be in for the happy ending!

ABOUT THE AUTHOR

MARISA BENNETT is the author of the national bestseller *Fifty Shades of Pleasure*. Her work has appeared in *Cosmopolitan*, *Allure*, *Penthouse*, and *HuffPost*, among others, and her best-selling sex guides have been sold worldwide and translated into more than a dozen languages. She lives with her husband in Minnesota.